The Art of Body Contouring

Edited by Alexandro Aguilera

Published in London, United Kingdom

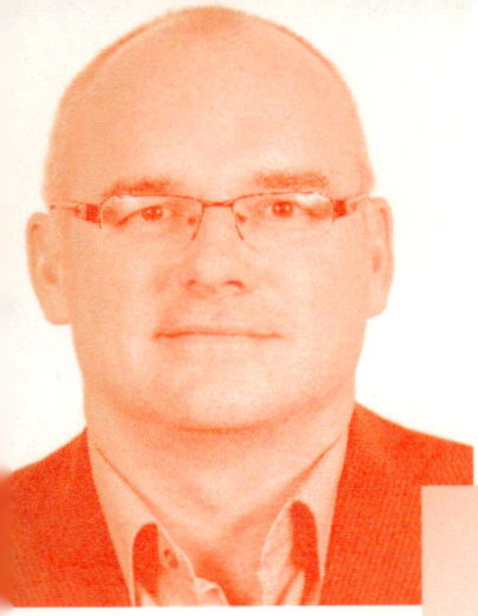
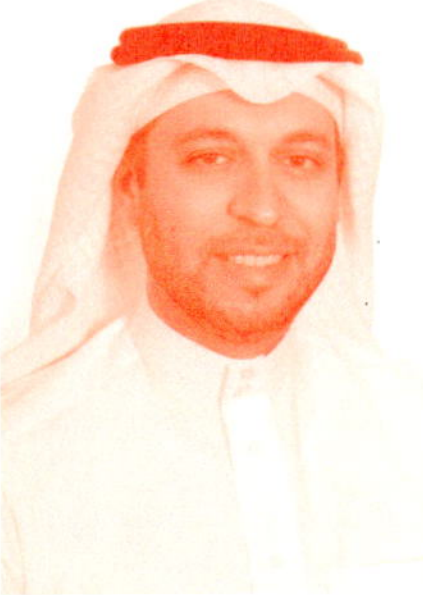
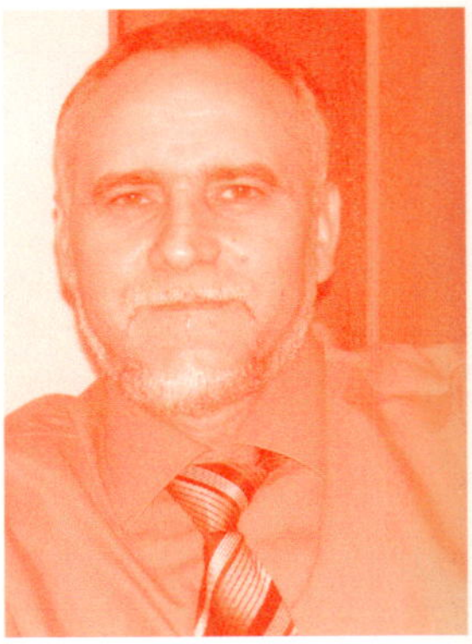
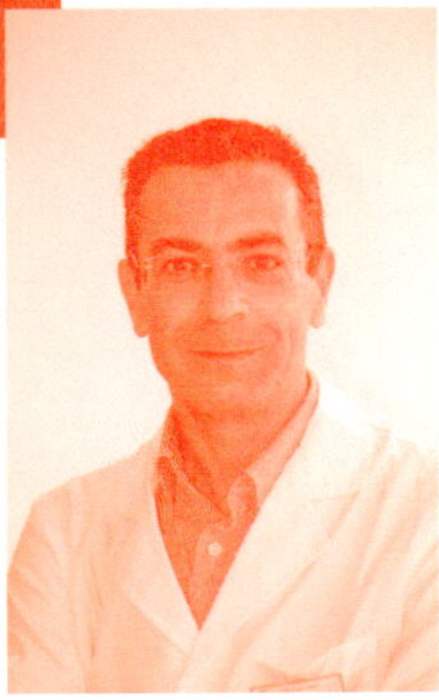
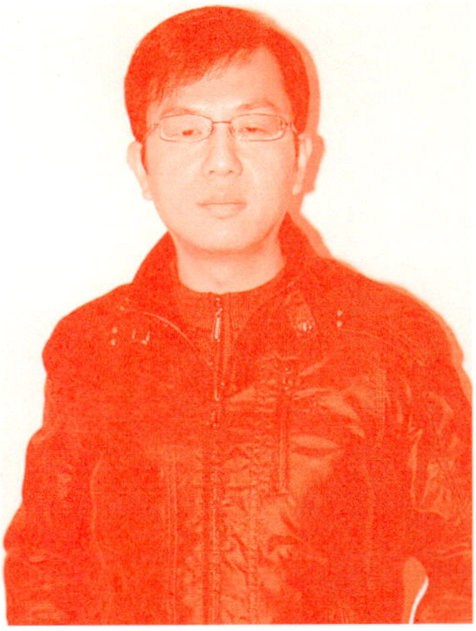
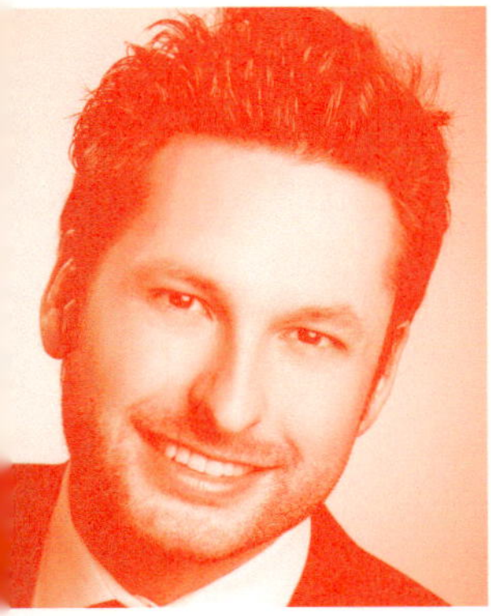
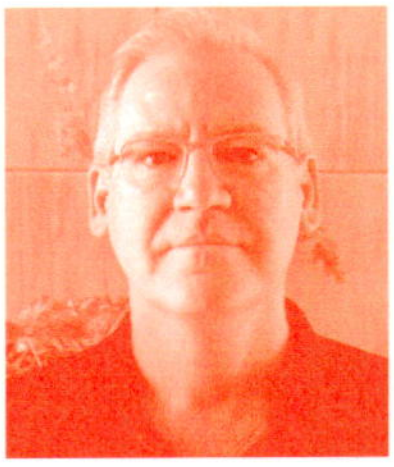

IntechOpen

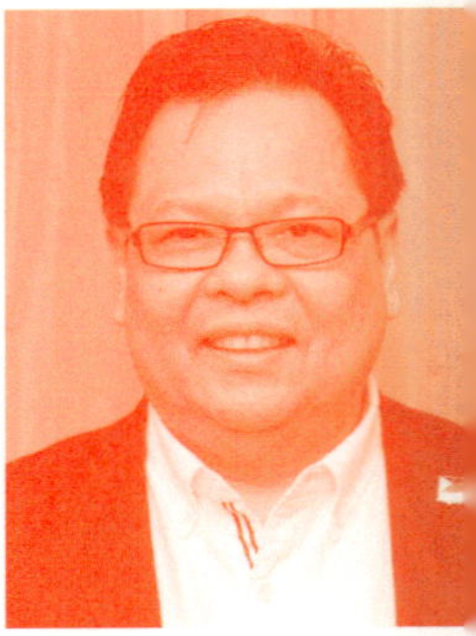
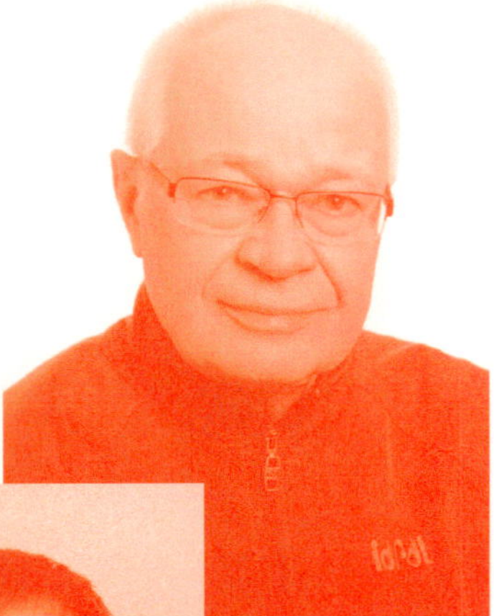
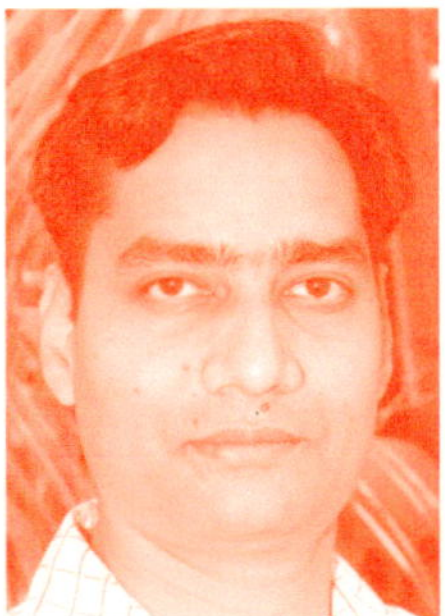
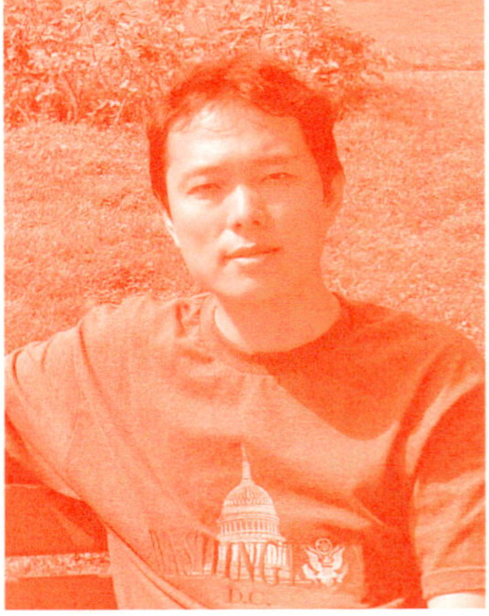
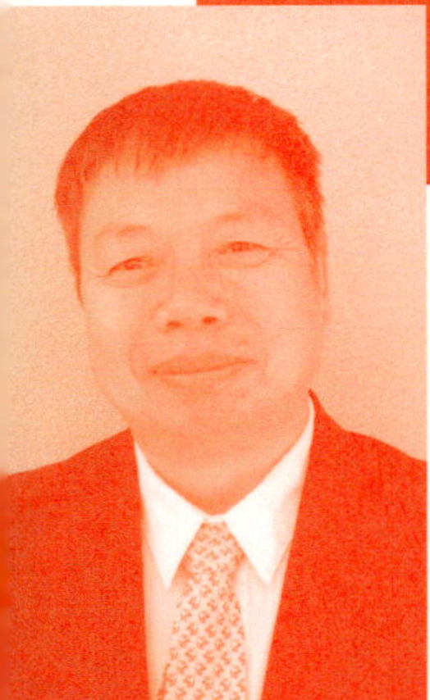
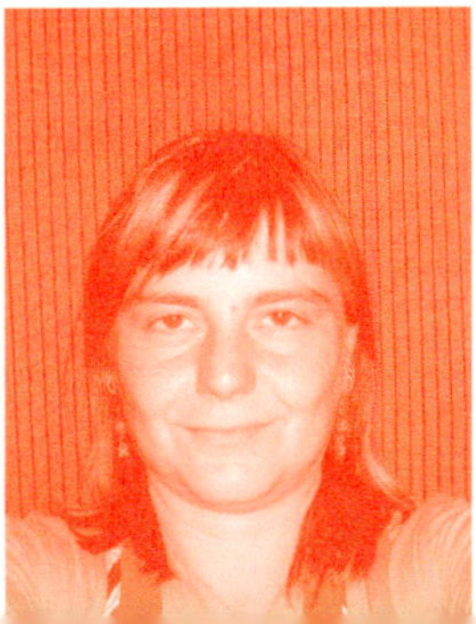

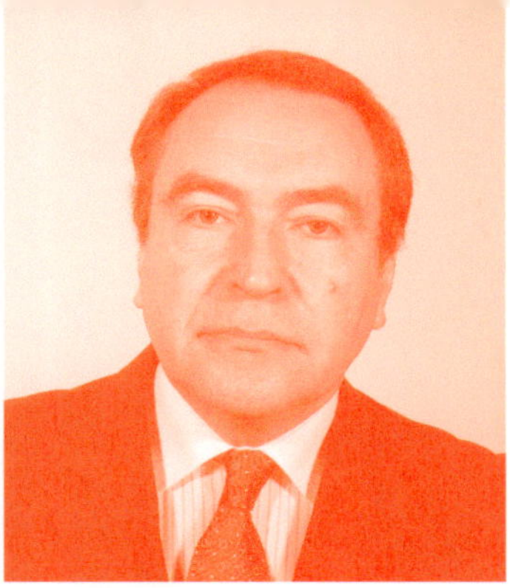
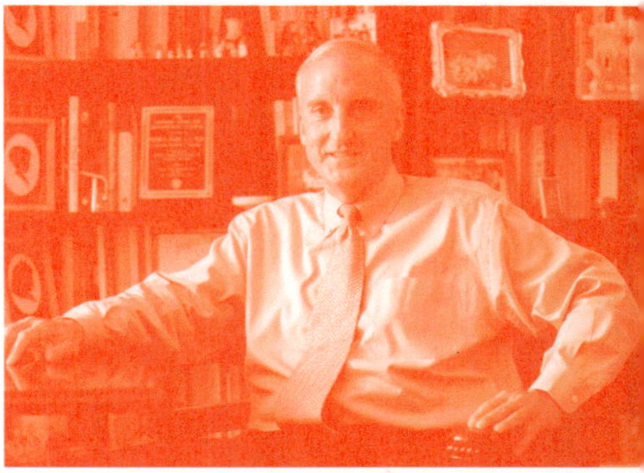
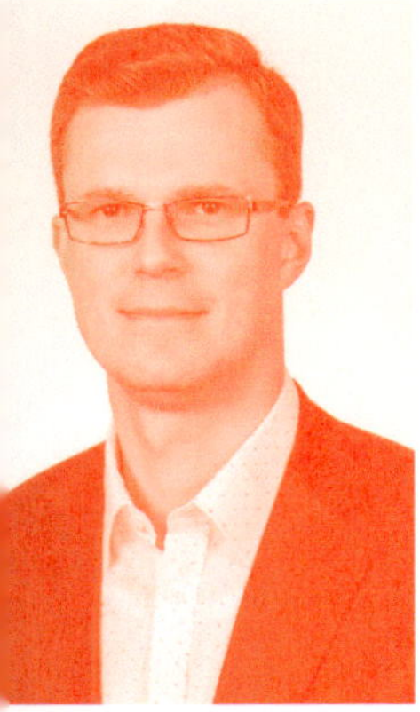
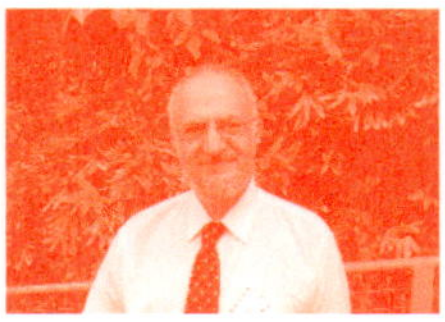
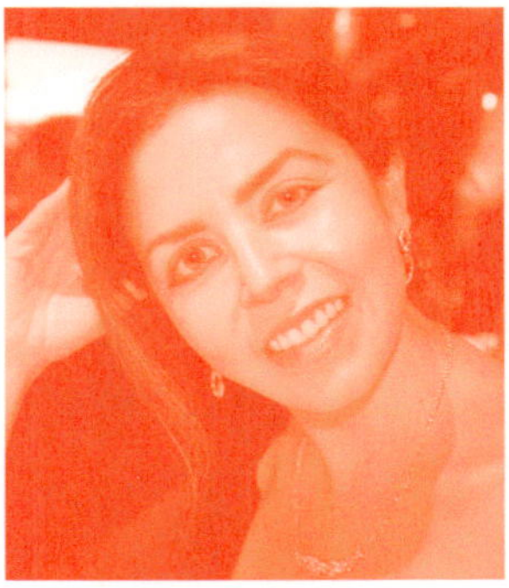

Supporting open minds since 2005

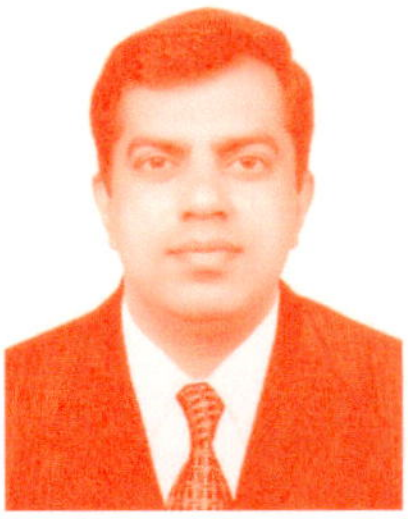
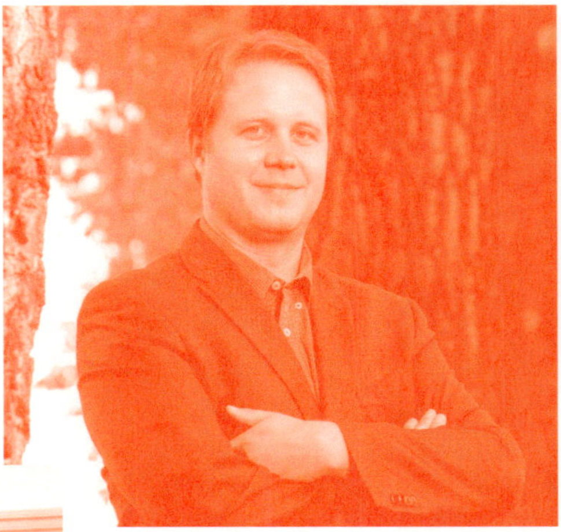
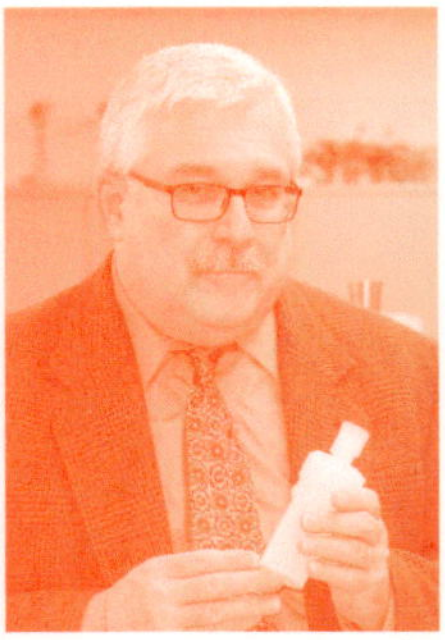
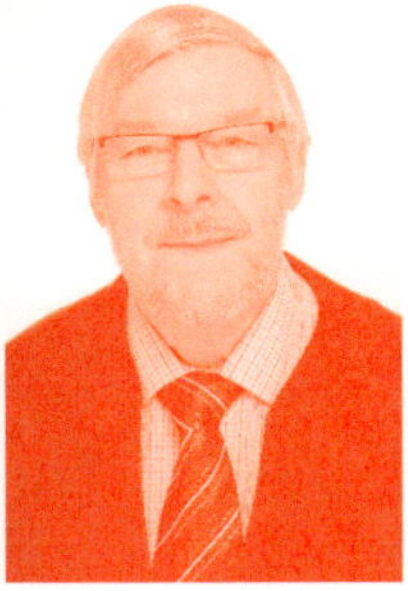
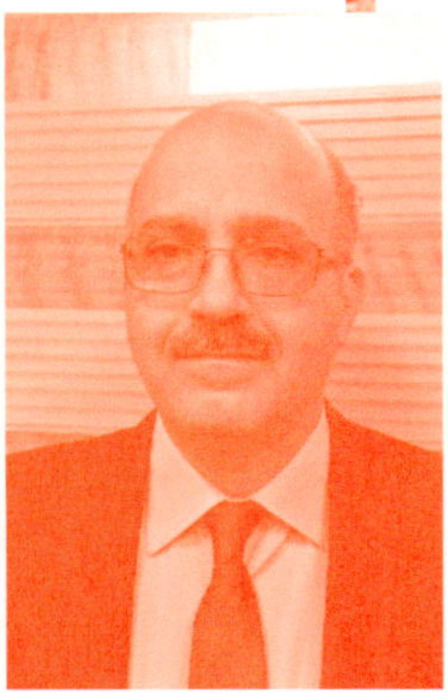
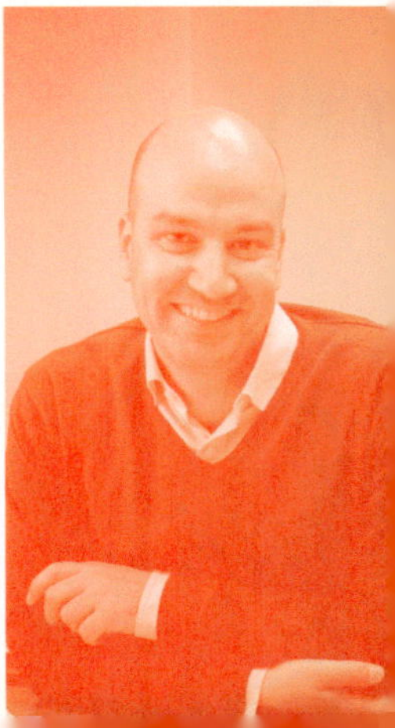
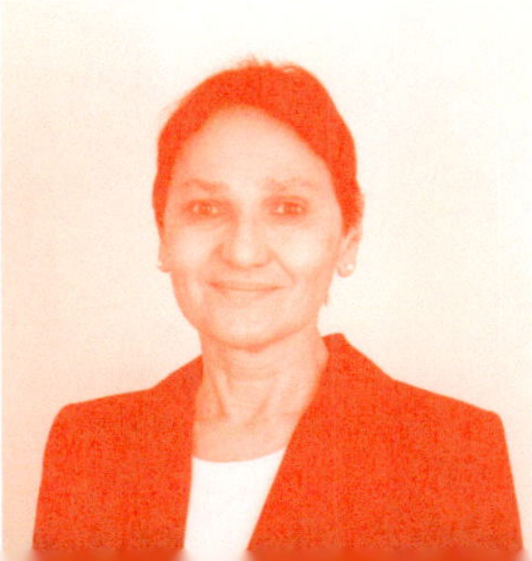

The Art of Body Contouring
http://dx.doi.org/10.5772/intechopen.77653
Edited by Alexandro Aguilera

Contributors
R. Stephen Mulholland, Yueh-Bih Tang, Shihheng Chen, Yo-Shen Chen, Diane Duncan, Alberto Di Giuseppe, Saverio Di Giuseppe, Federico Giovagnoli, Diana Ronconi, Angelo Cuzalina, Armando Retana, Landon McLain

First published in London, United Kingdom, 2019 by IntechOpen
IntechOpen is the global imprint of INTECHOPEN LIMITED, registered in England and Wales, registration number: 11086078, The Shard, 25th floor, 32 London Bridge Street
London, SE19SG – United Kingdom
Printed in Croatia

British Library Cataloguing-in-Publication Data
A catalogue record for this book is available from the British Library

Additional hard and PDF copies can be obtained from orders@intechopen.com

The Art of Body Contouring
Edited by Alexandro Aguilera
p. cm.
Print ISBN 978-1-78984-195-4
Online ISBN 978-1-78984-196-1
eBook (PDF) ISBN 978-1-78984-184-8

For EU product safety concerns:
IN TECH d.o.o., Prolaz Marije Krucifikse Kozulić 3, 51000 Rijeka, Croatia,
info@intechopen.com or visit our website at intechopen.com.

Meet the editor

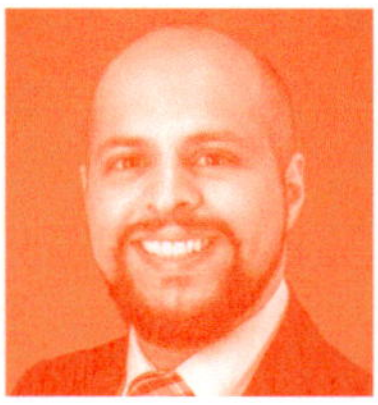

Dr. Alexandro Aguilera is a plastic and reconstructive surgeon and a faculty member of the Department of Plastic and Reconstructive Surgery at the National Institute of Pediatrics in Mexico City, Mexico. He is board certified by the Mexican Board of Plastic, Aesthetic, and Reconstructive Surgery. He has a fellowship in hand surgery and another one in facial palsy and peripheral nerves certified by the National Autonomous University of Mexico. He is part of the Educational Committee of the Mexican Association of Plastic Surgeons and has participated in numerous manuscripts, poster presentations, and books. He has contributed to several national and international plastic and reconstructive surgery meetings.

Contents

Preface

Body contouring surgery is one of the most common procedures performed by plastic surgeons worldwide. As the world advances, new technologies have been developed in all areas of medicine, and aesthetic surgery is no exception. New procedures and new technologies are being applied in our field, so it is mandatory for us to know how to use them and what are their main indications and possible results, so we can routinely apply them to our patients. Body contouring surgery is a very passionate field that demands careful planning and flawless execution. This is why we have gathered a group of clinicians and scientists with vast experience in body contouring surgery to discuss breast and body contouring surgery as the main objectives in this book.

The book is divided in two sections. Section 1 is called Breast Reshaping and it includes two chapters. In Chapter 1 Prof. Tang-Yueh-Bih discusses some of the most common procedures in breast surgery, special considerations during surgery, and postoperative care. In Chapter 2, MD Cuzalina Angelo and collaborators walk us through the process of simultaneous mastopexy and breast augmentation. Section 2 is called Abdominal and Gluteal Contouring. This section includes four chapters. In the first three, Dr. Duncan Diane, Mullholand R. Stephen, Dr. Di Giussepe Alberto, and collaborators review some of the most recent technologies (helium-driven plasma radiofrequency, BodyTite, and Vaser Body Sculpting) that are being applied in body contouring surgery, as well as their indications, how these technologies work, and what results can be expected. Finally, in Chapter 4, MD Cuzalina Angelo and collaborators help us understand how to create an ideal buttock, discussing the use of implants, lifting, or fat grafting.

I dedicate this work to my family: mom, dad, sister and wife. They are the greatest pillars I have in my life, and the ones that have made me what I am now—a responsible, honest, thirsty-for-knowledge man, who never gives up on anything. Thank you for your support and for being a source of inspiration. I also want to thank my mentors and colleagues for pushing me very hard day by day to achieve my goals. Last but not least, I want to thank my patients, because without them none of this would have been possible. Thank you all very much.

Dr. Alexandro Aguilera
Plastic and Reconstructive Surgeon,
Chief of Hand and Peripheral Nerve,
Department of Plastic and Reconstructive Surgery,
National Institute of Pediatrics,
Mexico City, Mexico

Section 1

Breast Reshaping

Chapter 1

Breast Recontouring

Yueh-Bih Tang, Shihheng Chen and Yo-Shen Chen

Abstract

The breast is an important structure of the human body in terms of function and esthetics. Derangements in breast mount—breast form/volume/profile/silhouette and nipple-areolar complex—size/shape/nipple projection are all concerns for not only females but also males. Simply esthetic problems of breasts encompass hypoplasia, atrophy, displacement of nipple-areolar complex, widened areola, redundant nipple, breast ptosis, macromastia, etc. Congenital anomalies of breast—Poland syndrome, pectus excavatum, pectus carinatum, etc.—all need to be taken care for restructuring of the body contour. Nowadays, breast cancer of different stages may need different reconstruction modality. Postmastectomy breast reconstruction is another big issue for plastic surgeons. This chapter on breast recontouring will address on every specific kind of breast contour disorders and imperfection, along with individualized strategies of refining, restoring, and reconstruction approaches.

Keywords: breast, recontouring, reshaping, reconstruction

1. Augmentation of breast

1.1 Augmentation of breasts with implants

1. A 34-year-old lady with breast hypoplasia received augmentation of breasts (275 ml on both sides) (**Figures 1–3**) [1].

2. A 38-year-old lady with atrophy of breasts after breast feeding received augmentation of breasts with 300 ml gel implant on each side (**Figure 4**).

3. A 26-year-old lady with hypoplasia of breasts; right side is a little smaller. Dark areola is also complained. After breast augmentation with gel implants, 200 ml in each side, areolar hyperpigmentation was greatly alleviated (**Figures 5** and **6**).

1.2 Augmentation of breasts with fat graft injection

1. A 25-year-old unmarried lady wished to have a more prominent breast profile; aspiration of abdominal fat for lipofilling of breasts 150 ml for each side was performed (**Figures 7–9**).

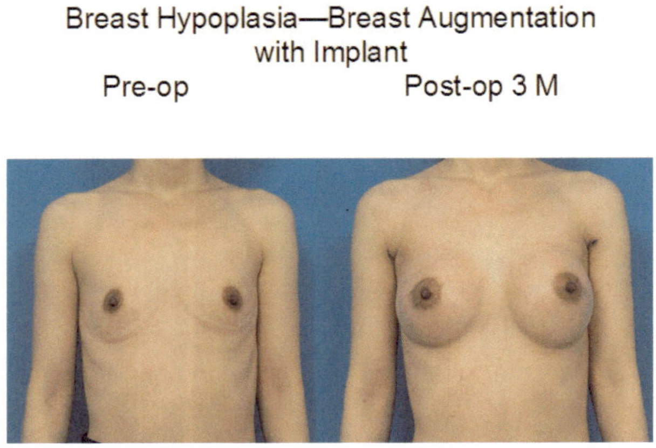

Figure 1.
Front view; left, pre-op; right, post-op; after breast augmentation with 275 ml gel breast implants.

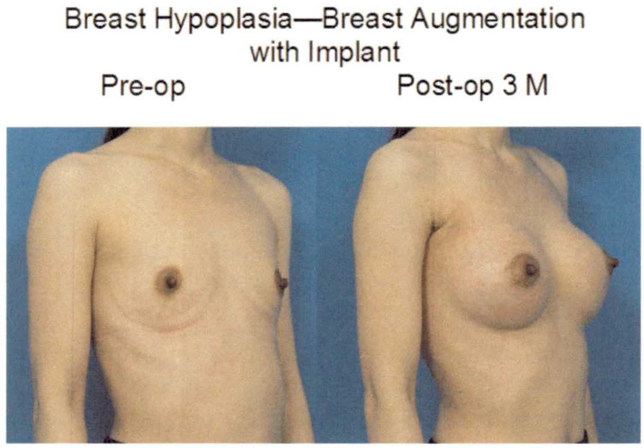

Figure 2.
Three-quarter view; left, pre-op; right, post-op.

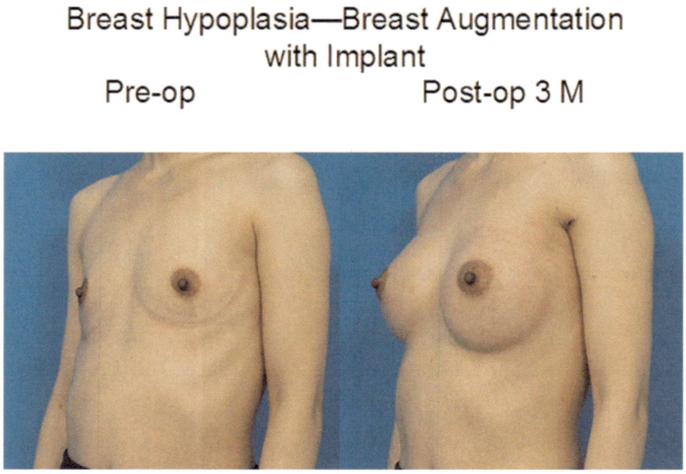

Figure 3.
Three-quarter view; left, pre-op; right, post-op.

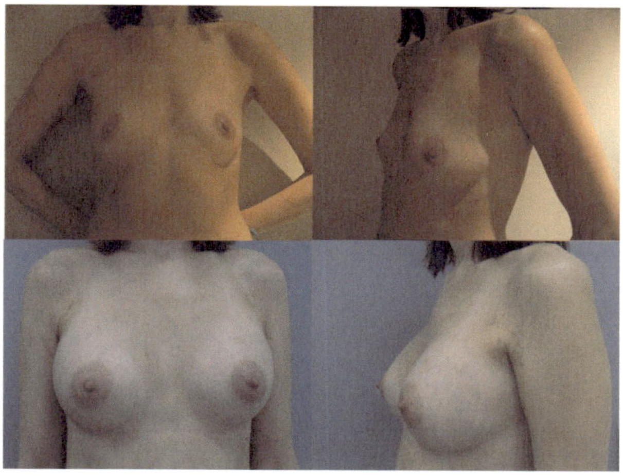

Figure 4.
Breast atrophy. Upper row, pre-op; lower row, breast augmentation with 300 ml gel implants at both sides.

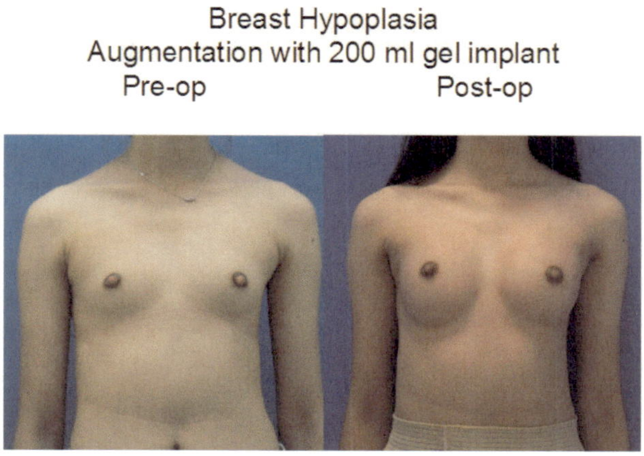

Figure 5.
Left, pre-op; right, post-op.

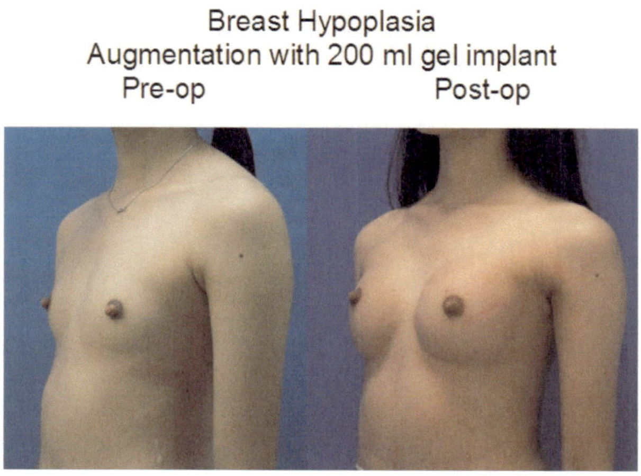

Figure 6.
Three-quarter view. Left, pre-op; right, post-op.

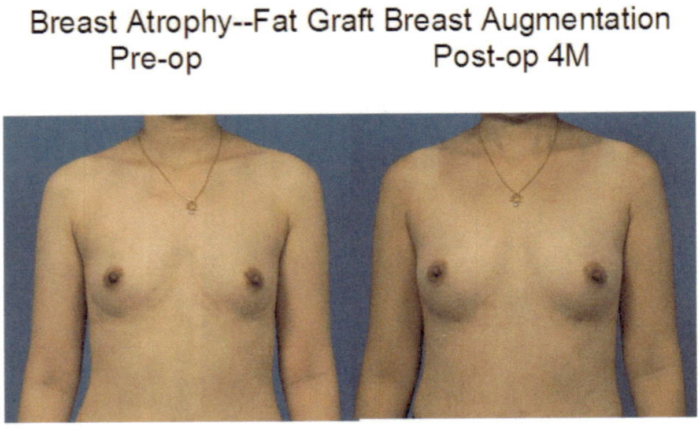

Figure 7.
Front view. Left, pre-op; right, 4 months post-op.

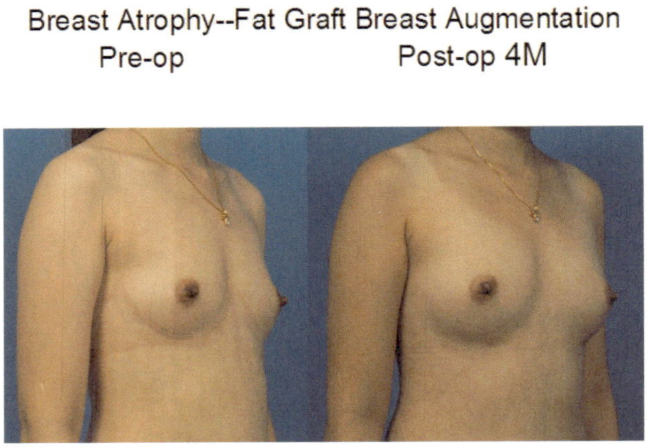

Figure 8.
Three-quarter view; left, pre-op; right, 4 months post-op.

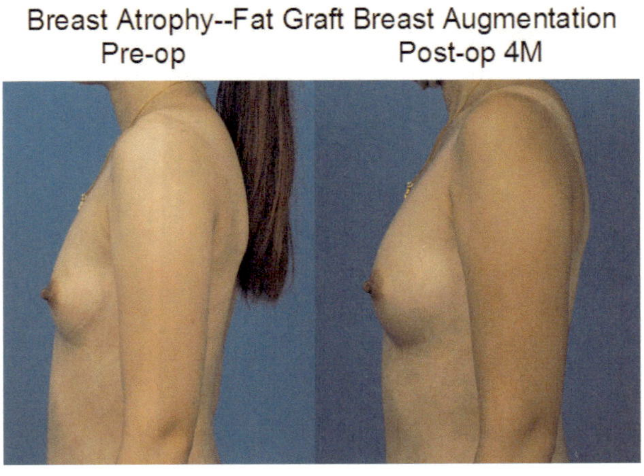

Figure 9.
Lateral view; left, pre-op; right, post-op.

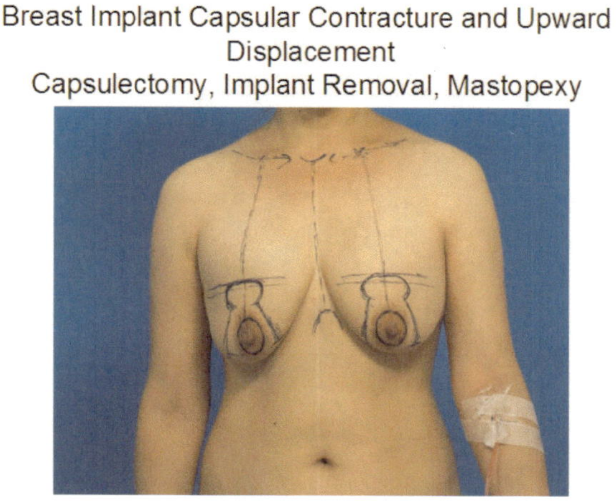

Figure 10.
Pre-op, upward displacement of augmented breasts with capsular contracture resulting in ptosis of breasts and displacement of nipple-areolar complex.

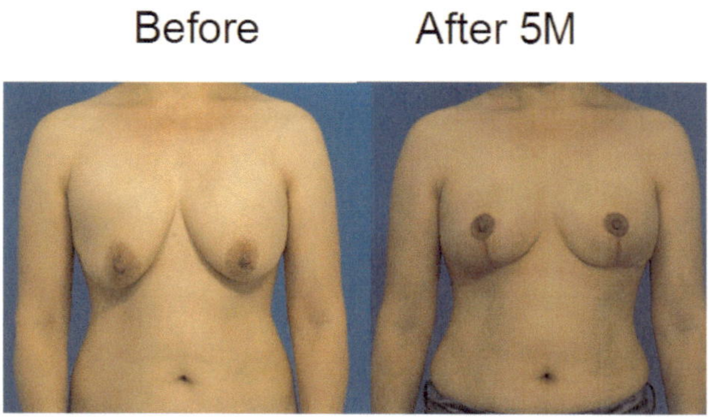

Figure 11.
Front view; left, pre-op; right, post-op.

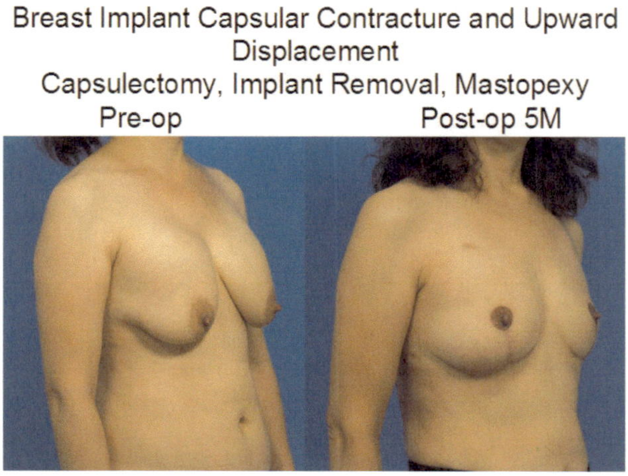

Figure 12.
Three-quarter view; left, pre-op; right, post-op.

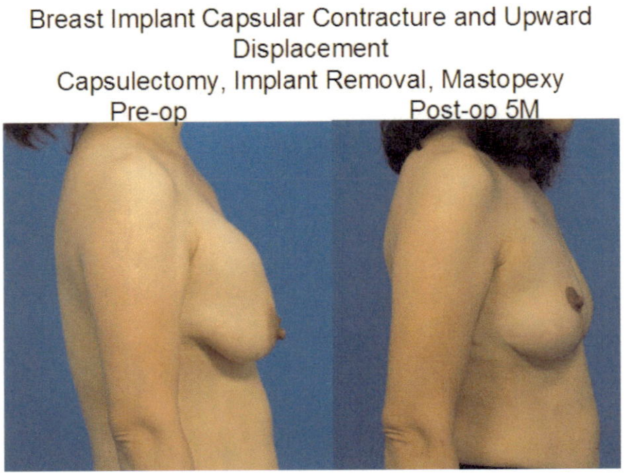

Figure 13.
Lateral view; left, pre-op; right, post-op.

2. A 43-year-old lady with upward displacement of augmented breasts with capsular contracture [2] resulting in ptosis of breasts and displacement of nipple-areolar complex.

She received removal of breast prostheses and surrounding capsules with mastopexy and reduction and reposition of nipple-areolar complex (**Figures 10–13**).

2. Reduction of hypertrophic breasts

1. A 20-year-old young lady, suffered from bilateral macromastia and received reduction of breasts with inferior pedicle technique (**Figures 14–16**) [3, 4].

2. A 41-year-old lady, augmentation of breasts at lower pole with gel implant and reduction with elevation and refinement of nipple-areolar complex (**Figures 17–19**).

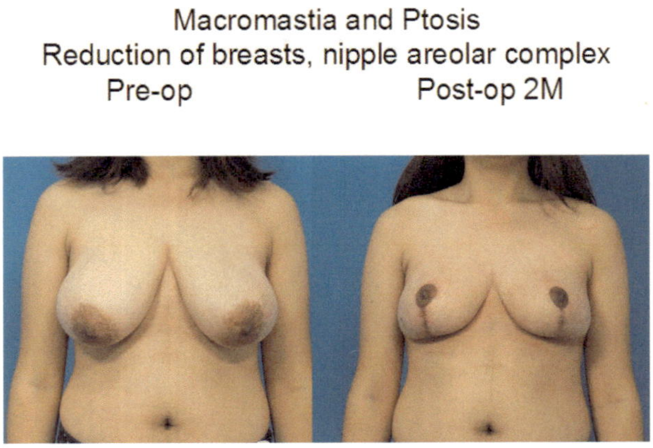

Figure 14.
Macromastia. Front view; left, pre-op; right, post-op.

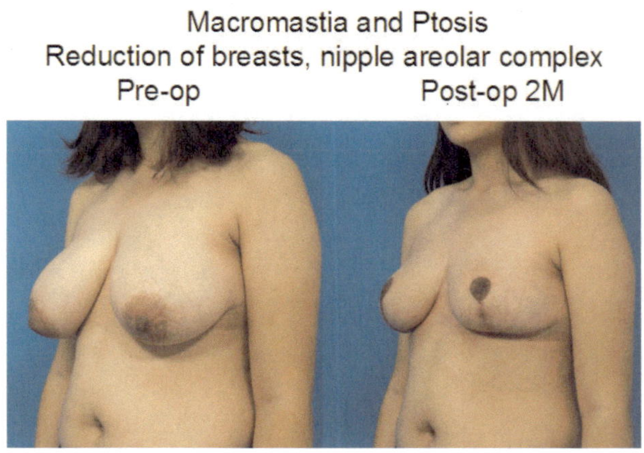

Figure 15.
Macromastia. Three-quarter view; left, pre-op; right, post-op.

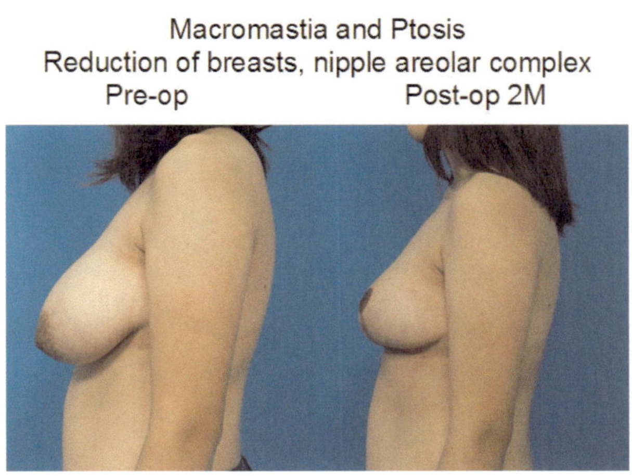

Figure 16.
Macromastia. Lateral view; left, pre-op; right, post-op.

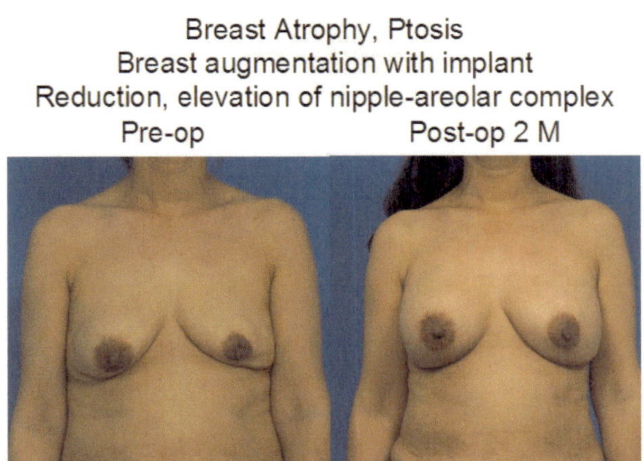

Figure 17.
Front view; left, pre-op; right, post-op.

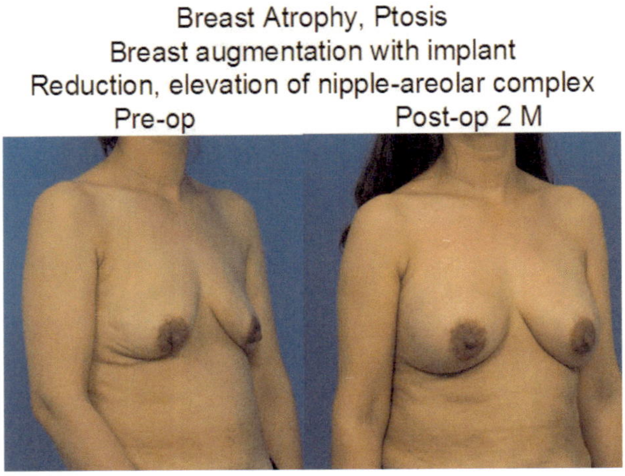

Figure 18.
Three-quarter view; left, pre-op; right, post-op.

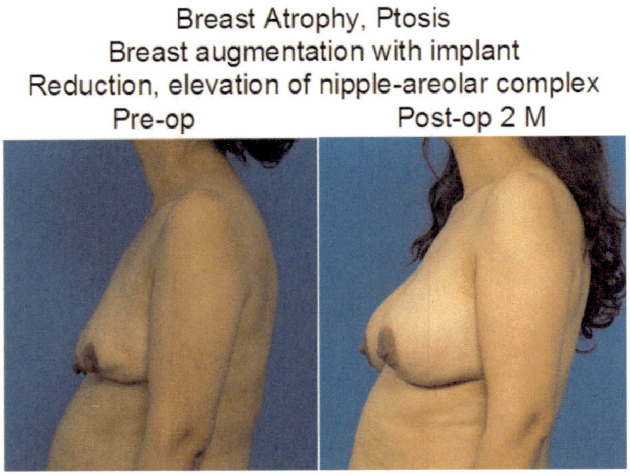

Figure 19.
Lateral view; left, pre-op; right, post-op.

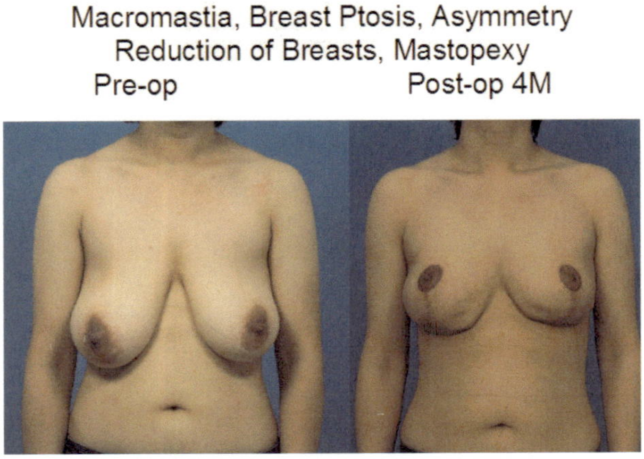

Figure 20.
Macromastia; left, pre-op; right, post-op.

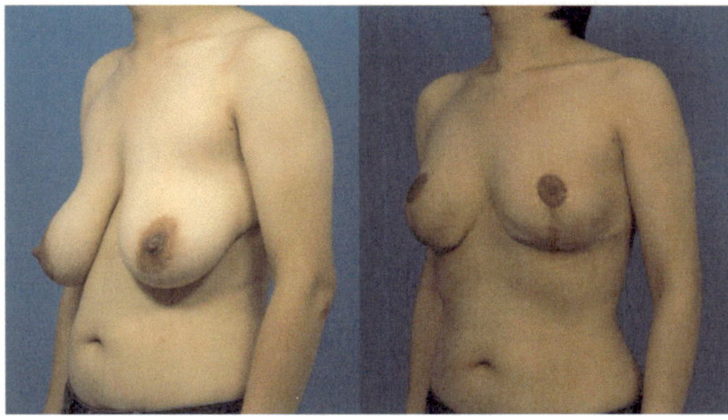

Figure 21.
Three-quarter view; left, pre-op; right, post-op.

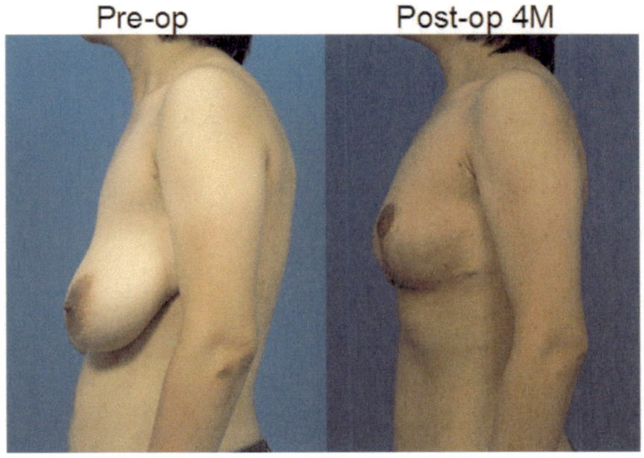

Figure 22.
Lateral view of macromastia and breast ptosis. Left, pre-op; right, post-op.

3. A 26-year-old young lady suffered from macromastia, which became breast ptosis and asymmetry after weight reduction. She received reduction of breast, mastopexy, and correction of breast asymmetry (**Figures 20–22**).

3. Mastopexy

1. A 57-year-old lady, with breast atrophy, ptosis, and significant breast asymmetry, left side more ptotic [5].

Mastopexy with dissecting medial and lateral flaps from the underlying breast tissue was brought together with upward mobilization of the nipple-areolar complex to build up more esthetic and symmetric breasts. The operation was carried out under local anesthesia (**Figures 23** and **24**).

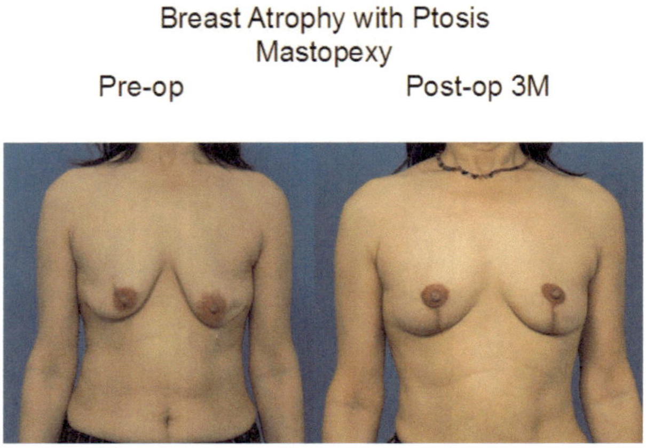

Figure 23.
Atrophic and ptotic breasts with significant asymmetry and disfigurement of nipple-areolar complex. Front view; left, pre-op; right, post-op.

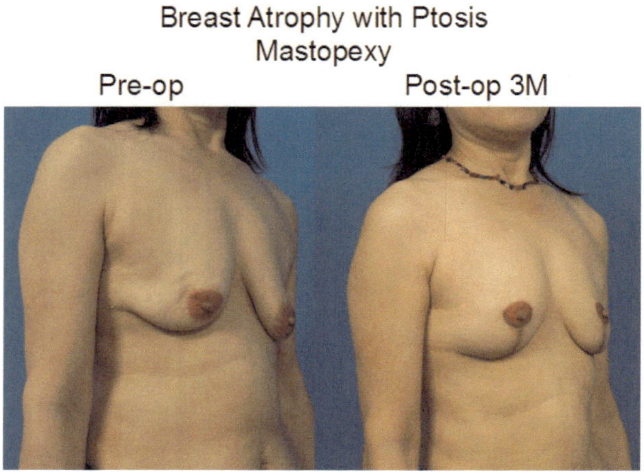

Figure 24.
Atrophic and ptotic breasts with significant asymmetry and disfigurement of nipple-areolar complex. Three-quarter view; left, pre-op; right, post-op.

4. Postmastectomy breast reconstruction

Nowadays, breast cancer patients are increasing, and different breast cancer treatment modalities are evolving, which may result in miscellaneous breast deformities, asymmetry, and disfigurements [6–9].

The patients may suffer from breast deformities, asymmetries, radiation injuries, loss or deformities of nipple-areolar complex, scar contracture, or even lymphedema of the affected side upper extremity.

Breast cancer of different stages may need different reconstruction modality. Postmastectomy breast reconstruction is another big issue for plastic surgeons.

1. This 38-year-old lady had modified radical mastectomy on her right breast. She received postmastectomy breast reconstruction 3 years later. Transverse

rectus abdominis myocutaneous flap [6, 9] was harvested from lower abdomen to reconstruct the right breast defect. The photo showed the breast figure 25 years after operation (**Figure 25**).

2. Twenty-eight-year-old lady with right side post-modified radical mastectomy received secondary breast reconstruction with free DIEP flap [9], followed by nipple-areolar reconstruction (**Figure 26**).

3. This 38-year-old patient received partial mastectomy followed by radiotherapy at left breast for breast cancer, resulted in a contracted and deformed breast [10]. The patient felt embarrassed with the breast asymmetry. Therefore she received differential augmentation of the breasts with gel implant (Mentor Memory gel) (right side 250 ml, left side 300 ml) (**Figures 27–29**).

4. This 51-year-old lady suffered from breast asymmetry and capsular contractures at both breasts [2], s/p breast cancer surgery and reconstruction with implants. The problems included nipple-areolar complex enlargement at right side, deficient areola at left side, and hardened breast at right side, which were corrected with nipple areolar sharing from right side to left side, change of breast implant size with capsulectomy, and differential augmentation (**Figures 30–32**).

5. This 37-year-old lady received left side partial mastectomy with irradiation at medial lower quardrant, resulting in significant breast deformity and asymmetry [10]. Her right breast was atrophic and ptotic. Therefore differential mastopexy of right breast and left breasts were performed, intending to achieve symmetricity of the breasts (**Figures 33–35**).

6. Chest wall deformity due to pectus excavatum [11–14] is corrected with "revascularization of turnover sternum," which is a definitive treatment for intractable funnel chest [15].

Intractable funnel chest in this 16-year-old young adult was treated with revascularization of the turnover sternum. The sternum and costal composite tissue were

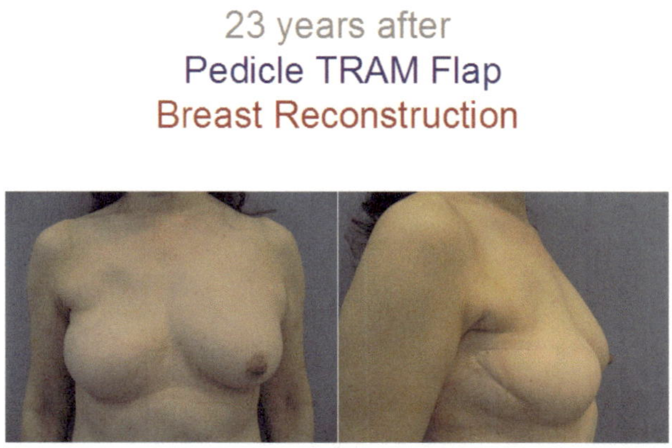

Figure 25.
Twenty-five years after postmastectomy breast reconstruction with pedicled transverse rectus abdominis myocutaneous flap.

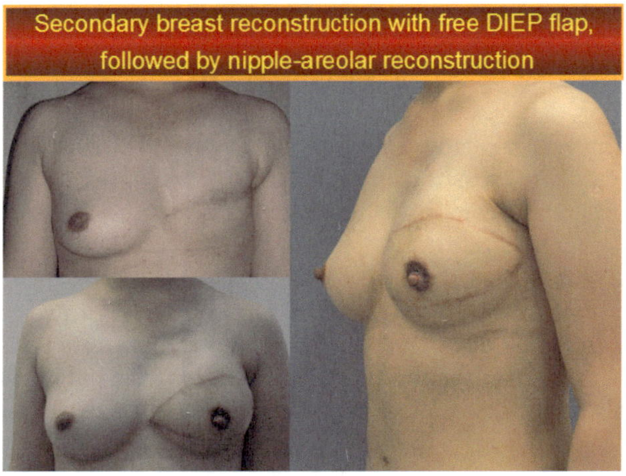

Figure 26.
Secondary breast reconstruction with free DIEP flap, followed by nipple-areolar reconstruction.

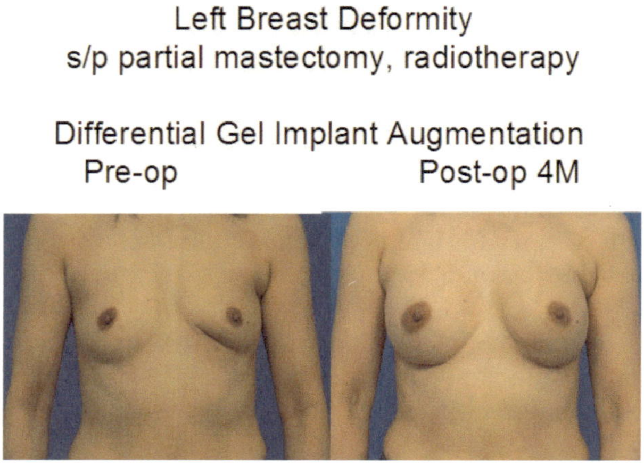

Figure 27.
Front view. Differential augmentation of the breasts with gel implant (Mentor Memory gel) (right side 250 ml, left side 300 ml). Left, pre-op; right, post-op.

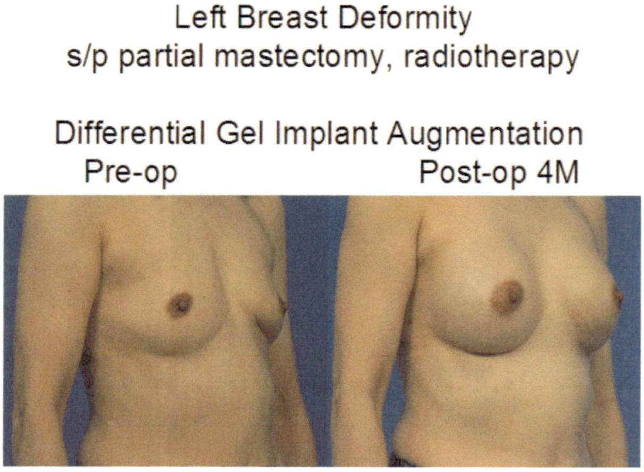

Figure 28.
Right three-quarter view. Differential augmentation of the breasts with gel implant (Mentor Memory gel) (right side 250 ml, left side 300 ml). Left, pre-op; right, post-op.

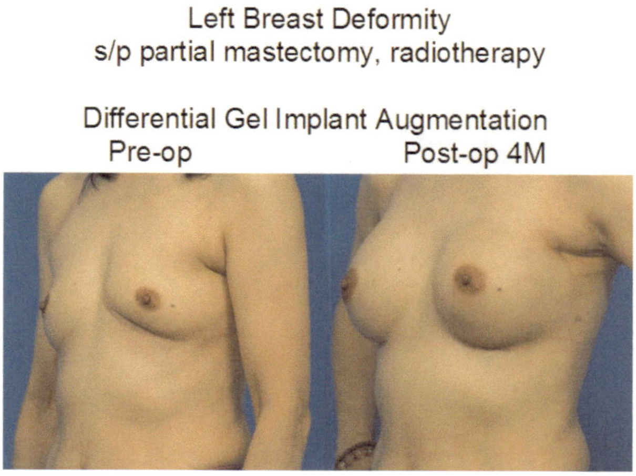

Figure 29.
Left three-quarter view. Differential augmentation of the breasts with gel implant (Mentor Memory gel) (right side 250 ml, left side 300 ml). Left, pre-op; right, post-op.

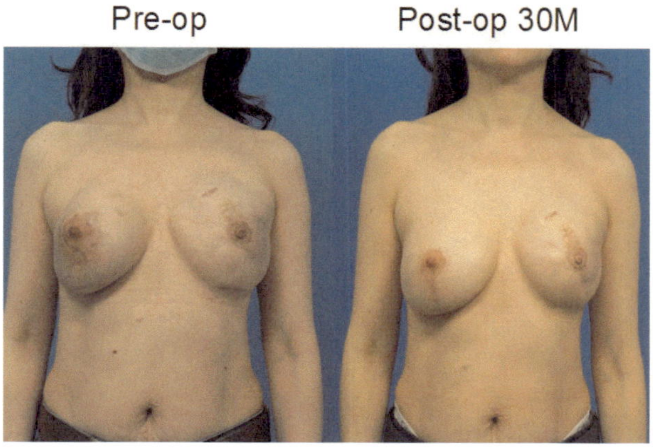

Figure 30.
Mastopexy, capsulectomy, change of prosthesis at right breast and capsulectomy, change of prosthesis, and areolar graft at left breast. Left, pre-op; right, post-op. 2.5 years.

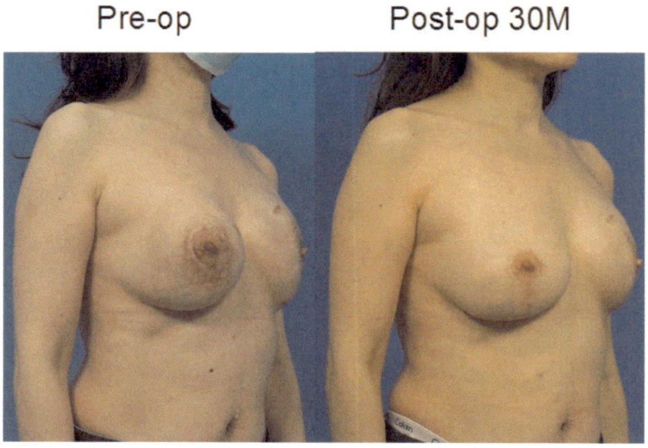

Figure 31.
Release of scar contracture with differential augmentation and nipple areolar sharing. Mastopexy at right breast. Right three-quarter view; left, pre-op; right, post-op.

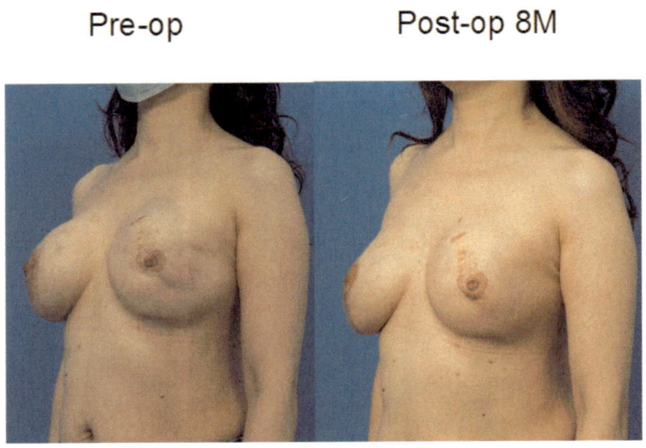

Figure 32.
Release of scar contracture with differential augmentation and nipple areolar sharing. Left three-quarter view; left, pre-op; right, post-op.

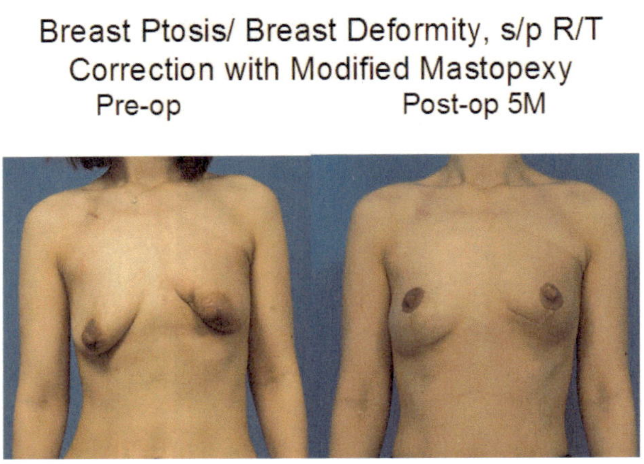

Figure 33.
Left, ptosis of right breast; deformity of left breast after partial mastectomy with R/T; left, pre-op; right, right breast corrected with mastopexy; left breast with modified mastopexy with subsequent fat graft.

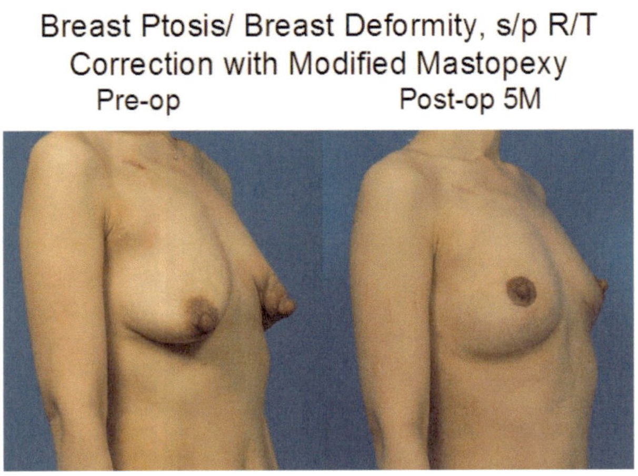

Figure 34.
Correction of right breast with mastopexy.

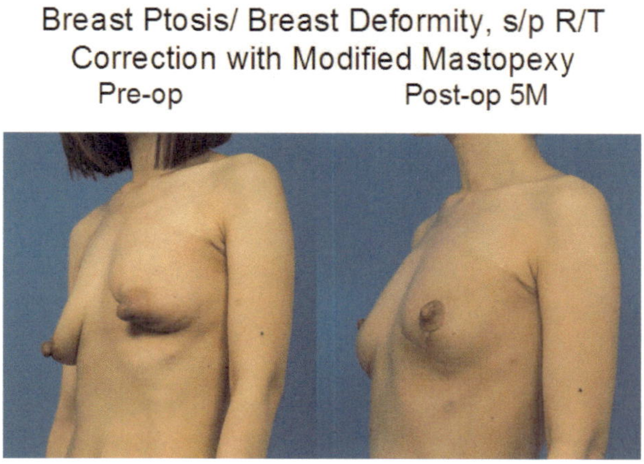

Figure 35.
Deformity of left breast after partial mastectomy with R/T, corrected with modified mastopexy with subsequent fat graft. Left, pre-op; right: Post-op. 5 months.

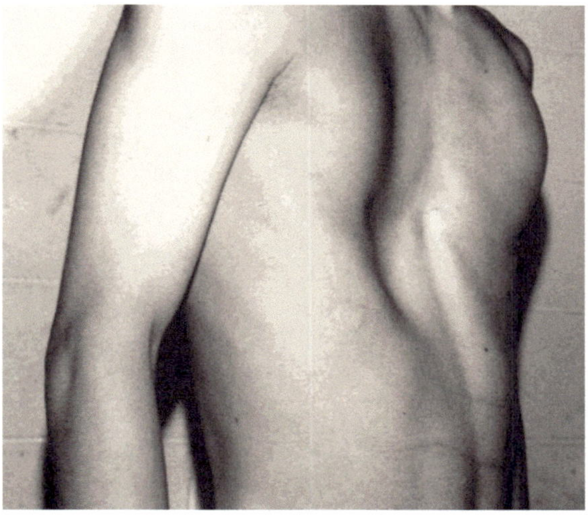

Figure 36.
Intractable funnel chest.

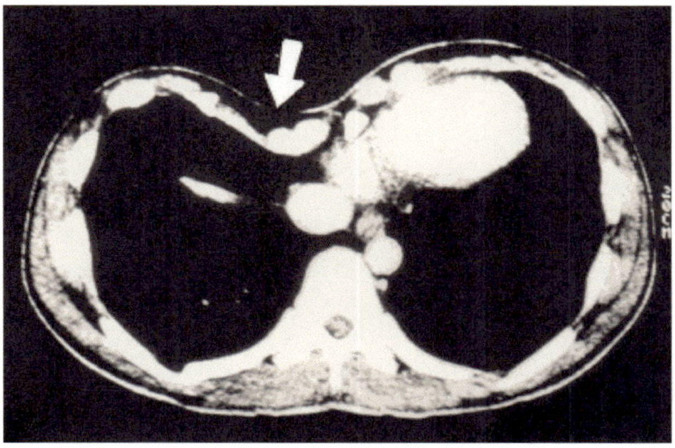

Figure 37.
CT showed compression of sternum on heart.

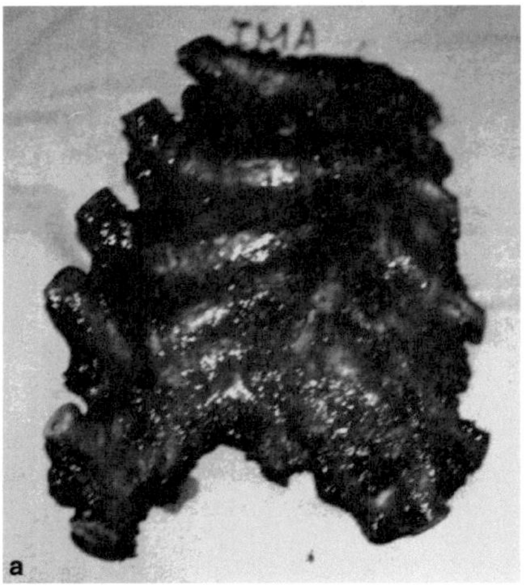

Figure 38.
Resected sternal block.

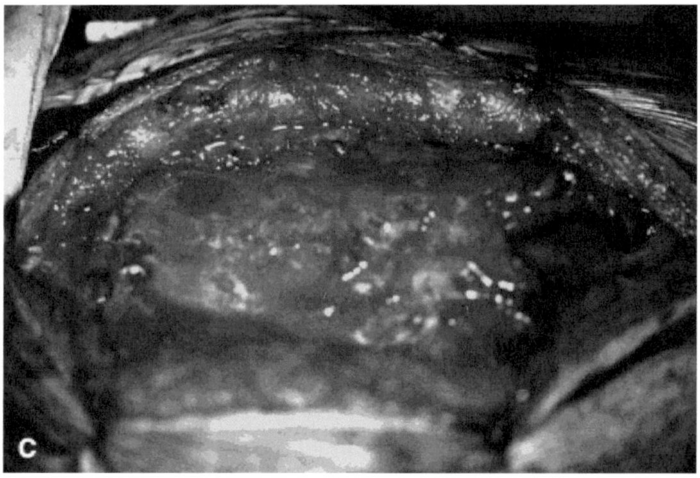

Figure 39.
Sternal turnover with revascularization.

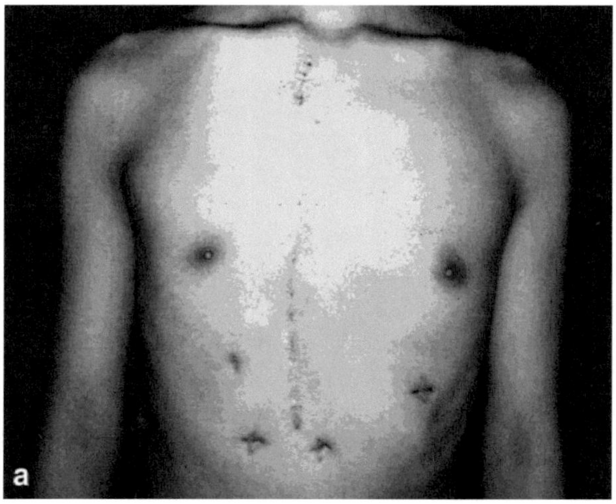

Figure 40.
Post-op front view.

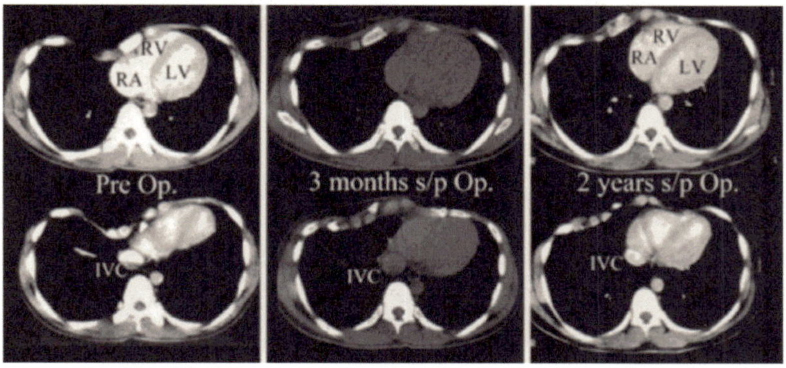

Figure 41.
Sequential CT follow-up showed definitive improvement of function, stability, and configuration of reconstructed sternum.

resected at the outskirt of the depressed area. Special attention was paid to the dissection of the vascular pedicle at both sides of the internal mammary vessels. The recipient vessels at one side were left long, so were the donor vessels at the other side. A segment of the rib at the exit of the recipient internal mammary vessels had to be removed to accommodate the vessels and to facilitate vascular anastomosis. Vascular anastomosis was accomplished with loupes (Keeler, sixfold magnification). Revascularization of the turnover sternum was performed successfully without vascular compromise. The patient recovered well with much improved physical condition. Postoperative three-dimensional computed tomographic (CT) scan revealed increment of thoracic cage volume for 9–17%. A follow-up CT scan 2 years later revealed even more improved thoracic cage expansion (**Figures 36–41**).

5. Gynecomastia

1. This 19-year-old young man had bilateral gynecomastia and out-projecting nipple, which made him feel embarrassed. Subcutaneous mastectomy with liposuction via tiny intra-areolar incision approach can achieve flatness of the breasts without leaving conspicuous scar (**Figures 42** and **43**).

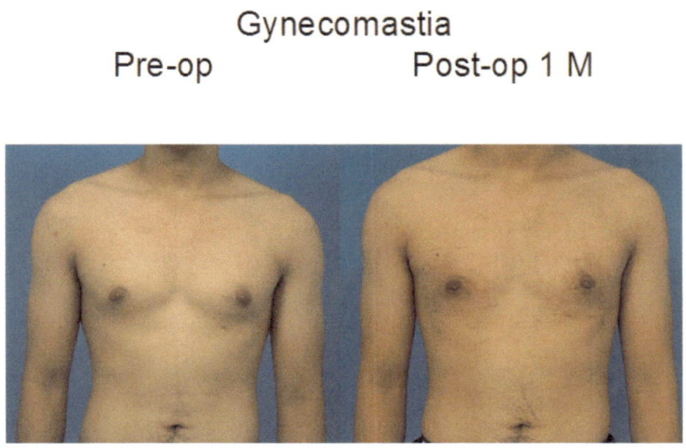

Figure 42.
A 19-year-old young man received correction of gynecomastia, showing flattening of breasts and bilateral nipple-areolar complex. Left, pre-op; right, 1 month post-op.

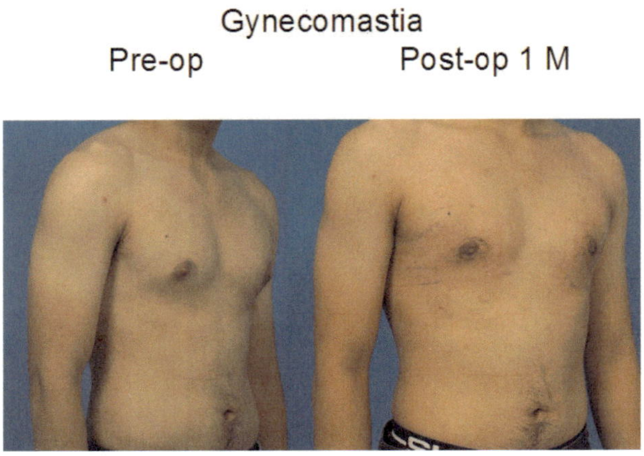

Figure 43.
A 19-year-old young man received correction of gynecomastia, showing flattening of breasts and bilateral nipple-areolar complex. Three-quarter view; left, pre-op; right, 1 month post-op.

6. Discussion

Breasts and forechest are important structures in esthetics and function in the human body [16]. Pursuing for a presentable breast and forechest contour has always been a goal for people. Imperfection at these specific areas is a common concern that brought to plastic surgeons.

This chapter introduces many kinds of breast problems, from simple to intriguing, with in-depth solutions. The breast with its unique role in esthetics and function brings about beauty and sorrow in a woman's lifelong journey.

The problems are:

1. Breast asymmetry

2. Breast volume—atrophy, and hypertrophy

3. Breast form disfigurement

4. Breast tissue and its enveloping skin incompatibility—breast ptosis and significant asymmetry

5. Deformity and displacement of nipple-areolar complex—in size, shape, length, and color

Breast cancer-associated complications:

1. Mastectomy-modified radical mastectomy.

2. Partial mastectomy

3. Total mastectomy

4. Subcutaneous mastectomy

5. Loss of nipple-areola complex

6. Radiation contracture

7. Radiation necrosis

8. Breast deformity

9. Scar contracture

10. Breast asymmetry

11. Chest wall deformity

12. Lymphedema at the afflicted upper extremity

Refinements in breast shape involve thorough evaluation for not only the inherent problem but also the status of the counterpart breast shape and form.

The nipple-areola complex is also an important esthetic unit that should be taken into consideration as a whole, which encompasses the size, form, length, color, etc.

Breast cancer surgery/radiation treatment [10] may create deformity, scar contracture, loss of nipple-areola complex, chest wall tightness, or even recurrence, radiation necrosis, infection, and cardiac tamponade of the severely afflicted individuals [10].

Reconstructions of the breast cancer surgery/treatment-associated problems involve placement of implant, with differential augmentation or reduction mammaplasty/mastopexy at the contralateral side. Nipple-areolar reconstruction can be elaborated with nipple areola sharing from the contralateral side, or by using local flap, followed by full-thickness skin graft and diced cartilage graft to create areola. The implant breast reconstructions are suitable for skin-sparing mastectomy patients.

Transverse rectus abdominis myocutaneous flap and free deep inferior epigastric perforator flap breast reconstruction are options for those with skin deficiencies or secondary reconstructions.

Choice of reconstruction modalities should consider the severity and general condition of the patient, expectation of the patients, and operation times that are desirable to the patients.

Pursuing excellence has been always the ultimate goal for breast surgeries and reconstructions.

7. Conclusion

Breast recontouring is a common request in the modern era. Introduction of the problems regarding this issue is well described and depicted in this chapter. With the advent of the current plastic and reconstructive surgery modality, almost all the problems can be solved to significantly improve the figure and life quality of the afflicted individuals. Pursuing excellence in plastic surgery and bringing excellence to life have always been our ultimate goals.

Author details

Yueh-Bih Tang[1,2*], Shihheng Chen[3] and Yo-Shen Chen[4]

1 Director of Center for Human Appearance, Far-Eastern Memorial Hospital, Banquio, New Taipei City, Taiwan

2 Department of Plastic Surgery, National Taiwan University Hospital, Taipei, Taiwan

3 Department of Plastic and Hand Surgery, Chang-Gung Memorial Hospital, Linko, Taiwan

4 Department of Plastic Surgery, Far-Eastern Memorial Hospital, Banquio, New Taipei City, Taiwan

*Address all correspondence to: phoebetang0103@gmail.com

References

[1] McGrath MG, Burkhardt BR. The safety and efficacy of breast implants for augmentation mammoplasty. Plastic and Reconstructive Surgery. 1984;**74**: 550

[2] Nelson GD. Complications from the treatment of fibrous capsular contracture of the breast. Plastic and Reconstructive Surgery. 1981;**68**:969

[3] McKissock PK. Reduction mammoplasty by the vertical bipedicle flap technique: Rationale and results. Clinics in Plastic Surgery. 1976;**3**:309

[4] Ribeiro L, Backer E. Inferior Based Pedicles in Mammoplasties. Georgiade NG, editor. Aesthetic Breast Surgery. Baltimore: Williams & Wilkins Company; 1983. p. 260

[5] Georgiade NG, editor. Aesthetic Breast Surgery. Baltimore: Williams & Wilkins Company; 1983. p. 260

[6] Hartrampf CR, Scheflan M, Black PW. Breast reconstruction following mastectomy with a transverse abdominal island flap anatomical and clinical observations. Plastic and Reconstructive Surgery. 1982;**69**:216

[7] Elliott LF, Hartrampf CR Jr. Tailoring of the new breast using the transverse abdominal island flap. Plastic and Reconstructive Surgery. 1983;**72**:887

[8] Georgiade GS, Riefkohl R, Cox E, McCarty KS, Siegler HF, et al. Long-term clinical outcome of immediate reconstruction after mastectomy. Plastic and Reconstructive Surgery. 1985;**76**:415

[9] Bostwick J. Breast reconstruction following mastectomy. Contemporary Surgery. 1987;**30**:16

[10] Bostwick J, Stevenson TR, Nahai F, Hester TR, Coleman JJ, Jurkiewicz MJ. Radiation to the breast. Complications amenable to surgical treatment. Annals of Surgery. 1984;**200**:543

[11] Crump HW. Pectus excavatum. American Family Physician. 1992;**46**: 173-179

[12] Hirayama T, Nozaki M, Wakamatsu S. A new surgical method for repair of funnel chest. Annals of Plastic Surgery. 1985;**14**:23-32

[13] Haller JA Jr, Kramer SS, Lietman SA. Use of CT scans in selection of patients for pectus excavatum surgery: A preliminary report. Journal of Pediatric Surgery. 1987;**22**:904-906

[14] Wada J. Sternal turnover. The Annals of Thoracic Surgery. 1974;**17**: 296-298

[15] TangChen YB, Chen SJ, Lee YC, Huang KF, Chen HC. Revascularization of turnover sternum: A definitive treatment for intractable funnel chest. Microsurgery. 1999;**19**:296-302

[16] McCarty KS Jr, Glaubitz LC, Thienemann M, Riefkohl R. The breast: Anatomy and physiology. In: Georgiade NG, editor. Aesthetic Breast Surgery. Baltimore: Williams & Wilkins Company; 1983. p. 1

Chapter 2

Simultaneous Mastopexy with Augmentation

Angelo Cuzalina and Landon McLain

Abstract

Simultaneous mastopexy and augmentation can be an extremely rewarding surgery for both patient and surgeon. However, it is one of most complex cosmetic surgical procedures with a high revision rate, relatively high complication rate and higher than average litigation rate. Trying to simultaneously adjust two breasts for a new submuscular implant pocket, new NAC position, new parenchymal arrangement, new infra-mammary fold (IMF) position, great symmetry, perfect amount of skin and fat removal, with great scars all while maintaining vascularity is no small task. A clear understanding of the optional procedures and variables involved when combining these techniques will significantly benefit the surgeon in obtaining safe and predictable results while limiting the vast majority of complications.

Keywords: mastopexy, breast augmentation, simultaneous breast lift and augmentation, revision breast surgery

1. Rationale

The ability to correct both breast ptosis and deflation is a critical component in any successful cosmetic breast practice. In most offices, the percentage of patients desiring correction of both the aforementioned deformities is significant if not a majority. Multiple factors lead to both ptosis and deflation, including pregnancy and lactation, weight loss and congenital abnormalities, any of which can ultimately result in descent of the nipple-areola complex (NAC) below the inframammary crease. This is usually accompanied by some degree of reduction in breast volume, leading to the desire for "larger and perkier" breasts which is a common request from the affected patient population. The required manipulation of these multiple components, the breast skin envelope, glandular area and position, NAC position and size, inframammary fold position and chest wall anatomy is what makes this procedure technically and strategically challenging. However, mastery of this combination procedure will yield far more dramatic and esthetic results then either augmentation or mastopexy alone [1, 2]. The remainder of this chapter will be focused on helping the reader better understand both the obvious and subtle factors in performing this procedure in a reliable and predictable fashion with minimization of risks and complications. Simultaneous breast lift and augmentation carries a high litigation rate because the complication and revision rates are much higher than the majority of cosmetic surgeries. Trying to simultaneously adjust two breasts for a new submuscular implant pocket, new NAC position, new parenchyma arrangement, new infra-mammary fold (IMF) position, great symmetry, perfect amount of skin and fat removal, with great scars all while maintaining vascularity is

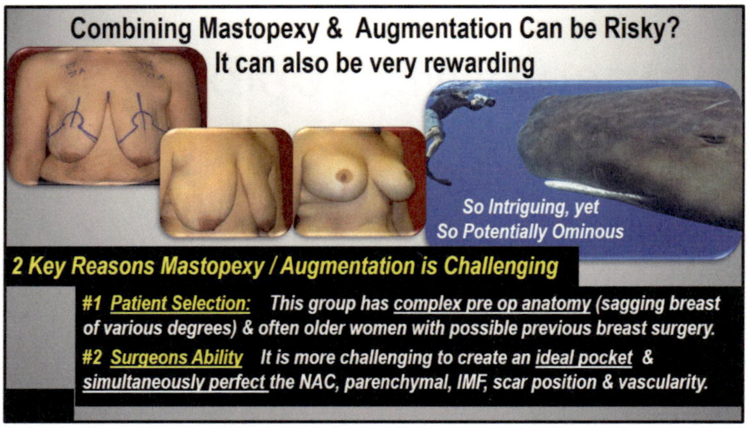

Figure 1.
Simultaneous breast lift and augmentation is extremely gratifying when it works well but carries a high litigation rate because it is a very challenging procedure and risk are relatively high for complication. Removing and tightening skin at the same time one increases volume of the breast with an implant by its nature risk nipple-areola complex (NAC) necrosis.

no small task. But, by improving so many issues of the ptotic breast, potential positive changes and patient's happiness can be wonderful and rewarding (**Figure 1**).

2. Options

Of course the basics of this procedure are some combination of augmentation with elevation of the NAC with varying degrees of skin/glandular excision. The simplest form would be a basic augmentation with a crescent lift of one or both areolae, while the more challenging case can require a large reduction/lift using an inverted T incision along with augmentation (**Figure 2**). In either case, the goal is to augment the breast volume and reposition the NAC into a more harmonious relationship with the breast implant while successfully managing the soft tissue envelope and glandular area. In our opinion, the mastopexy portion of the procedure allows one to manipulate and idealize the breast tissues, in other words *match,* the breast tissues around

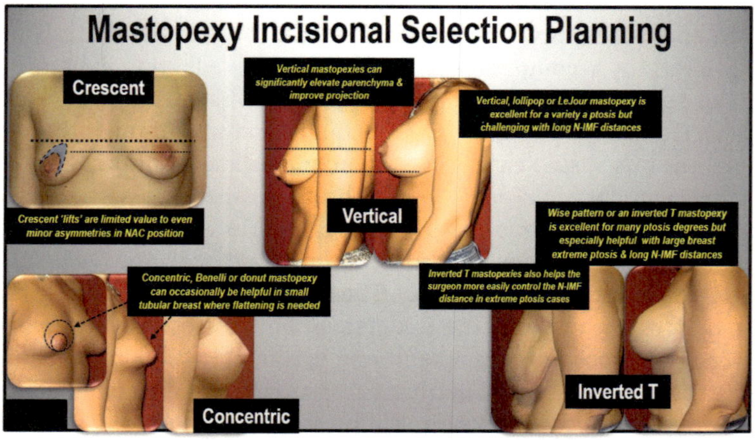

Figure 2.
Many incisional options exist for mastopexy but all breasts are different along with patient desires. The basic four options shown above are the crescent, concentric, vertical and inverted T. The vertical and inverted T mastopexies are the most efficient choices for the majority of breast ptosis situations.

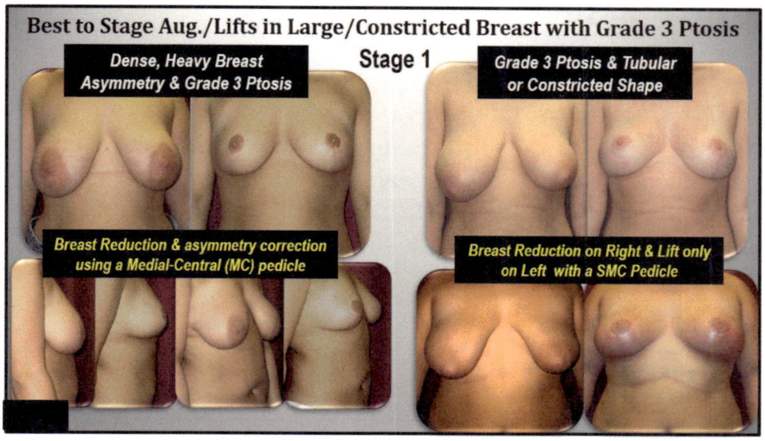

Figure 3.
The primary aim of staging is to avoid the devastating complication of ischemia and necrosis to the NAC. Extremely large breast with major ptosis as well as large tubular or constricted breast as shown are ideal for staging when a patient desires both mastopexy/reduction plus implants for a more "rounded" or "perky" appearance.

a well-placed and selected implant. However, one must consider limitations to both of the components of the surgery, which are stricter in combination than either in isolation. For example, a breast augmentation alone may allow use of larger implants, but when combined with a mastopexy, the volume of implant must often be limited to avoid undue stress on the resultant breast envelope as well as the arterial perfusion and venous drainage of the NAC. Despite using a smaller implant in certain situations to decrease vascular compromise, the breast implant dimensions should still come close to the base width of the breast. This may often require avoiding a higher profile implant in favor of a more moderate profile and smaller implant that still has the desired base width, particularly when more extensive mastopexy is required.

At this point it is worth noting that not all patients are good candidates for this procedure. If there is extreme laxity, desire for extremely large breasts, or large pedunculated or constricted breasts requiring major reduction and tissue rearrangement staging may be the better option. The primary aim of staging is to avoid the devastating complication of ischemia and necrosis to the NAC which is most at risk (**Figure 3**). Medical co-morbidities and prior surgery may also lead one to recommend staging in select cases as well, but for the majority of patients requiring increased breast volume and repositioning of the NAC and reduction of excess skin are better served by combining these procedures. This often allows a type of synergism from matching the breast envelope to a well-positioned and selected implant that can yield a dramatic and pleasing result while minimizing financial burden, as well as anesthesia and recovery times for the patient.

3. Pertinent anatomy

The mammary gland begins as an invagination ectoderm that forms a primary bud which results in the development of multiple secondary buds, usually 15–25. Approximately halfway through gestation the buds have lengthened and formed epithelial chords that extend into the chest wall and then begin to form the lactiferous ducts through lumenization. At birth the lactiferous ducts open into the mammary pits that elevate and form the nipple. Failure to do so results in an inverted nipple (2–4% of females). No further development occurs until puberty when hormonal stimulation triggers proliferation and enlargement of the glandular tissues as well as deposition of fat.

3.1 Surface anatomy

The variation in size and shape of the female breast is considerable. Typically, the breast extends from the 2nd or 3rd rib superiorly to the 5th or 6th rib inferiorly where the inframammary crease lies. Medially the breast starts from the sterna-costal junction laterally to the anterior axially spine and may extend to the middle axillary line with the axillary tail extending supero-laterally into the axilla proper [1]. Ideally, the breast should form a rounded and conical shape with the NAC situated at the apex. The NAC may be of varying size and pigmentation, but ideally the NAC should be roughly 1/3rd of the overall breast diameter and the nipple itself 1/3rd of the overall areolar diameter [2].

3.2 Glandular anatomy

15–25 Lactiferous ductules extend from the deep glandular regions toward the NAC, terminating as openings. Each ductule drains 15–20 lobules which is the functional unit of the breast gland where lactation occurs. The breast gland has no discrete fascia but does have fibrous thickenings scattered throughout the gland which extend from the muscular fascia toward the skin. These Cooper's ligaments provide scaffolding support to the glandular breast. The integrity of these ligaments can be compromised with aging, fluctuations in weight and breast size and pregnancy which may eventually contribute to breast ptosis. Recent anatomic studies have elucidated additional internal supporting structures. The inframammary crease ligament has been identified through cadaver dissection and contributes to a well-defined inframammary crease. It typically extends from the medial aspect of the 5th rib and laterally to the fascia of the 5th and 6th ribs [3]. The ligamentum suspensorium mammae extends from the clavicle down to the upper border of the breast and retromammary space and may explain the propensity of some females to develop ptosis while other do not, as it is well defined in some patients but indistinct in others [4, 5].

4. Innervation, lymphatics and blood supply

Sensory innervation is derived from cervical plexus, anteromedial and anterolateral intercostal nerve branches from the 3rd, 4th, 5th and 6th intercostal nerves as well as branches from the 2nd intercostal nerve. Of particular concern for surgeons is the innervation of the nipple, which has crossover innervation from 3rd to 5th nerves medial and laterally, but primarily derived from the 4th lateral cutaneous branch. This branch tends to run along the fascia of pectorals major before emerging to innervate the nipple from its posterior surface.

Most of the lymphatic drainage of the breast flows into the axilla through the external mammary nodal group, however additional drainage occurs through the medial, transpectoral and postdoctoral routes as well.

The internal mammary artery supplies the majority (approximately 60%) of the blood supply to the breast. Its branches pass through the intercostal muscles, from the 2nd through 5th ribs immediately lateral to the parasternal border. These coalesce once in the breast with additional contributions from lateral thoracic branches, pectoral branches from in internal thoracic artery and branches from the posterior intercostal arteries. Venous outflow occurs via an anastomotic plexus in the subcutaneous tissue immediately beneath and around the NAC. This plexus then drains peripherally via large subcutaneous veins that empty into intercostal and axillary veins as well as internal thoracic veins. Importantly, the largest and most reliable venous routes reside in the superomedial and inferior pedicles. Congestion of these routes and the subareolar plexus are usually the primary causes of NAC ischemia and necrosis in mastopexy procedures [1].

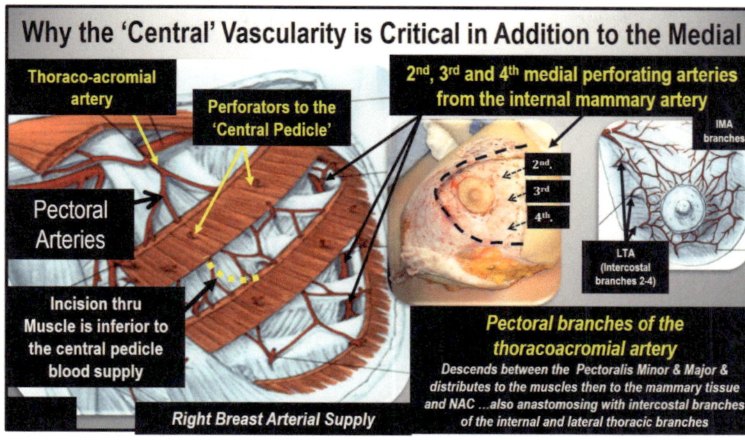

Figure 4.
The figure demonstrates the two major sources of blood supply to the Superomedial-Central (SMC) pedicle. The medial source from branches of the internal mammary artery and central component from the pectoral perforators. The 2nd medial perforator supplies the most superomedial area of the SMC pedicle. Maintaining all these sources during dissection produces a robustly vascularized pedicle.

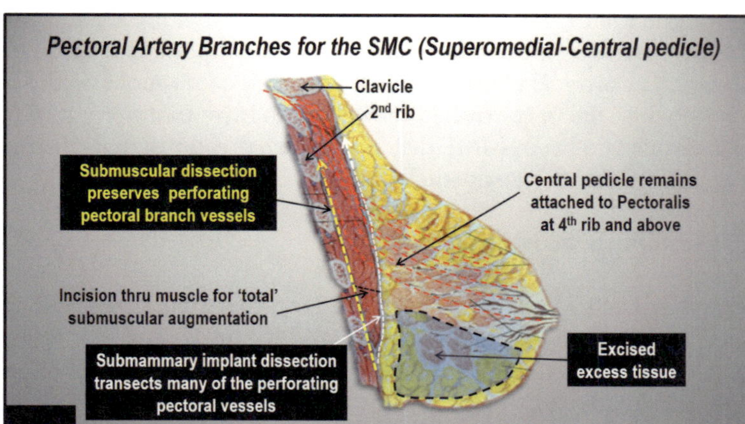

Figure 5.
The central component vascularization of the SMC pedicle is helpful when implant placement is submuscular. Submammary dissection transects most of the central perforators leaving only the medial perforators for blood supply to the NAC. The incision through muscle must be made just inferior to the central blood supply. Incision at the lateral pectoralis border can be used as well but does not work as well for obtaining a total muscular coverage of an implant.

4.1 Key point

The 2nd–4th medial perforating arteries from the internal mammary artery along with pectoral arteries branches from the thoracoacromial artery together supply the best blood supply to the NAC and is the primary reason the Superomedial-Central (SMC) pedicle is our pedicle of choice in the majority of combined mastopexy/augmentation cases (**Figures 4** and 5).

5. Incision options

As this chapter is focused on mastopexy with augmentation, we will primarily discuss vertical and Wise pattern mastopexy incision choices. Minimal attention will be afforded to crescent lift or periareolar (donut) mastopexy which have little major lifting benefit in most cases.

5.1 Crescent/circumareolar

The crescent lift has value mainly as a minor NAC elevation maneuver when one NAC is slightly higher than the other by 1–2 cm. It can help "level" out the position to match the other but has little to no lifting effect on the parenchyma. While the donut or circumareolar lift is best used for limited and isolated cases of a smaller tubular or severely constricted breast where flattening of the NAC may be desired. It is the authors' belief that the circumareolar lift yields undesirable results in the majority of cases and also has limited ability to manipulate the soft tissue envelope resulting in inadequate projection, poor scarring and lack of longevity.

5.2 Wise pattern/inverted T

This is the most commonly used mastopexy and reduction pattern in the United States and is similarly very popular when combined with augmentation. This can be based on multiple pedicles, with the inferior pedicle being the most preferred historically. However, other pedicles have gained popularity in recent years, particularly superior and medial pedicles. Although related, the skin excision pattern and glandular pedicle are separate components and each component should be selected based on thoughtful surgical planning. The horizontal component on the Inverted T incision is very beneficial in controlled the Nipple to Inframammary fold (N-IMF) distance in patients who have N-IMF distances much greater than 8–10 cm prior to surgery. It can be used with most pedicles and ptosis situations.

5.3 Vertical mastopexy/teardrop

Popularized by Lassus and LeJour and later modified by Findlay-Hall, the vertical mammoplasty traditionally seeks to avoid the horizontal scar relying on gathering excess inferior skin during closure and additional volume reduction is aided by liposuction inferiorly and laterally. Unfortunately, final breast shape can take many months to achieve and may still require skin excision inferiorly if puckering persists. The advantages that this technique offers are less incisional scarring, good projection, and this technique allows a versatile pedicle design. We feel the Superomedial-Central (SMC) pedicle is the most predictable and versatile pedicle due to more robust blood supply and venous drainage and this pedicle works very well with a vertical or inverted T mastopexy.

6. Pedicle options/implant location options

When combined with a central component, the superomedial pedicle has the most robust and unaffected blood supply during a combined mastopexy and augmentation procedure [6]. Hence, our pedicle of choice in the majority of mastopexy augmentations is the Superomedial-Central (SMC) pedicle. This majority of blood supply for this pedicle originates from the internal thoracic artery (via the internal mammary artery) that should be preserved using a SMC. The central component houses trans-pectoral perforators from the internal thoracic artery and medial mammary branches (**Figure 4**). This central component vascularization can only be maintained well when placing implants in a subpectoral or submuscular plane and are sacrificed with development of a subglandular pocket (**Figure 5**). This is an important consideration when selecting implant plane and in revision surgery when implants may have been placed in a subglandular fashion. For the aforementioned reasons, the authors almost universally use subpectoral or submuscular placement during the augmentation phase of the procedure. This is not only beneficial from a blood supply and venous drainage perspective, but also results in more soft tissue coverage of the implant and likely results in a decreased incidence of capsular contracture. An additional advantage is when utilizing a *total submuscular* plane, the elevated fibers of serratus and external oblique with their corresponding fascia are elevated partially to help cover the implant inferiorly and laterally to dissuade bottoming out and as a further barrier to the external environment and potential microbes should even a small wound dehiscence occur postoperatively (**Figure 6**). This is particularly important when capsular contracture exists above muscle and

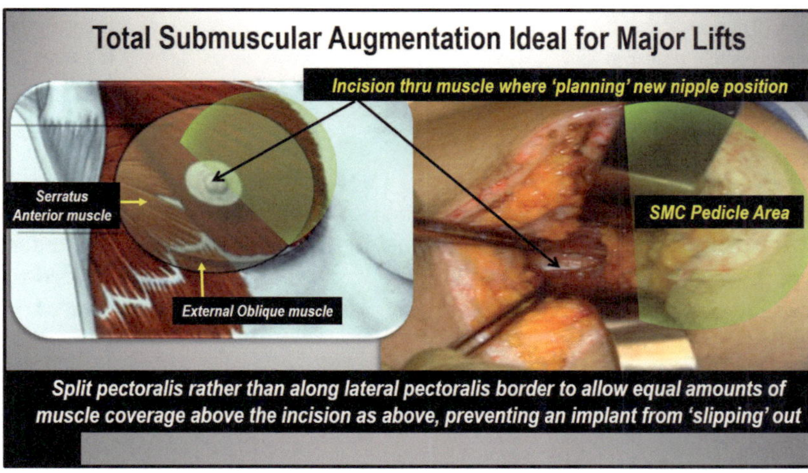

Figure 6.
The SMC pedicle allows for implant placement in a total submuscular location if the incision as shown is made immediately inferior to the central pedicle component that remain attached to the pectoralis major. Total coverage of a new implant gives protection of any incision breakdown and also prevents the implant from "slipping out" of the pocket especially when a submammary implant was simultaneously removed.

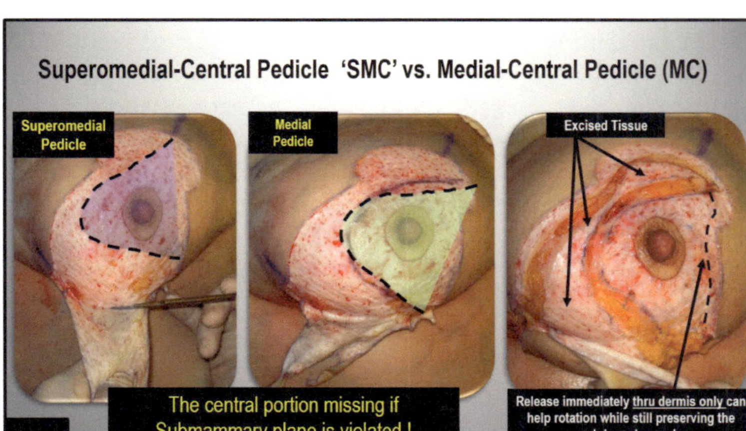

Figure 7.
While the SMC can be used in most ever breast ptosis situation, when the sternal notch to nipple (SN-N) distance becomes greater than 30 cm, a MC pedicle improves the arc of rotation to obtain proper NAC elevation with less kinking of the pedicle. Most of the same blood supply exists between a SMC vs. MC pedicle with the occasion loss of the 2nd intercostal in some medial pedicle situations.

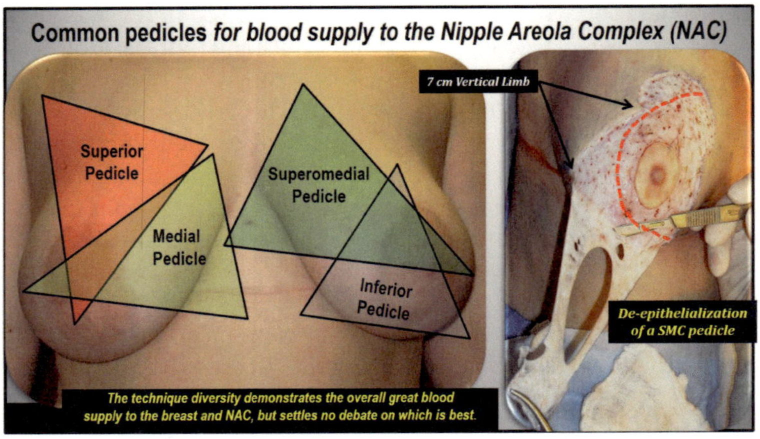

Figure 8.
The four most common pedicles as discussed and shown here have specific advantages and disadvantages. Regardless, the surgeon must make sure any of the four if used is treated gently and has an adequate base to allow proper drainage to and from the NAC.

a complete capsulectomy is performed and a new implant is immediately placed beneath muscle in a new pocket. In this situation, a subpectoral placement only will result in "slipping out" of the implant from the subpectoral position back into the above muscle pocket unless an acellular dermal matrix (ADM) is added to the inferior muscle edge. The total submuscular placement prevents implant slippage and avoids the need for an expensive ADM placement.

Although the SMC pedicle likely offers the most versatility and safety, this can be altered in select situations (**Figure 7**). For instance, a purely Medial-Central (MC) pedicle should be considered in cases of long pedicle length and greater degrees of ptosis (SN-N > 30 cm) such as some massive weight loss patients. This option allows for maintenance of the medial mammary and pectoral arterial branches while allowing an easier or better "arc of rotation" of the pedicle into its final position, without excessive kinking or tension on the pedicle [7]. In cases where the mastopexy component is fairly small and the degree of NAC elevation minor (only 2–3 cm), a purely superior-central (SC) pedicle can often facilitate easier transposition of the NAC into position [8]. A purely SC pedicle will gain some axillary artery contribution as well as some lateral and internal thoracic branches to the pedicle [9]. An inferior pedicle is rarely selected in certain staged procedures where the patient has a very long SN-N along with a relatively short N-IMF distance (**Figure 8**). Because the inferior pedicle bottoms out more than other pedicles, the vertical limbs of an inferior pedicle should be drawn close to 5 cm compared to a 7 cm length of vertical limbs for superior, medial or superomedial pedicles that have very limited stretching comparably.

7. Implant selection

The style and type of implant used is quite variable. This technique performs well regardless of implant style used assuming some common considerations. Saline or silicone implants are well suited for this procedure and their selection should be based on similar criteria one would use for augmentation alone typically. However, given that the implant plane is sub muscular, the incidence of rippling is less than with a subglandular plane. As previously mentioned implant size is critical. Utilizing very large implants can stress the mastopexy closure and lead to ischemia to the NAC. A more conservative approach to implant sizing is preferable and avoidance of excessively high profile implants can help to avoid wound complications. Although textured, anatomically shaped implants have gained popularity, it is the authors' opinion that usually, the smooth round implants perform best in combined mastopexy/augmentation surgery by removing the variable of rotational alignment intraoperatively required with the use of anatomically shaped implants.

8. Preferred technique

Operative sequence for the authors preferred technique differs from others in that the mastopexy is performed first and implant placement is performed prior to closure. Although, theoretically this could increase the risk of over resection of skin, this has not often been encountered with thoughtful skin marking/resection and implant selection. The primary advantage gained is the ability to place the implant in a total submuscular plane and more fully manipulate the skin and glandular elements of the procedure. It also can be challenging to estimate ideal implant position prior to the mastopexy when there is significant ptosis or asymmetry combined with the typical alteration of the inframammary crease that can occur during mastopexy. It is for these reasons that the mastopexy is initiated first followed by implant placement, then glandular manipulation as required and finally skin closure.

8.1 Marking

Mastopexy marking is performed with an indelible marker with the patient in upright or standing position for obvious reasons. A mastopexy template is beneficial and can facilitate symmetry. Either a Wise pattern or vertical pattern is marked with emphasis on positioning the NAC at or slightly above the inframammary crease. In cases where you may be unsure if a horizontal skin excision will be required it is advisable to mark the patient with a vertical excision plan (**Figure 9**). Minor horizontal excision can be done accurately and easily intraoperatively. However, most cases requiring any significant degree of skin resection or NAC elevation, are best served by Wise pattern excision which controls the nipple to fold

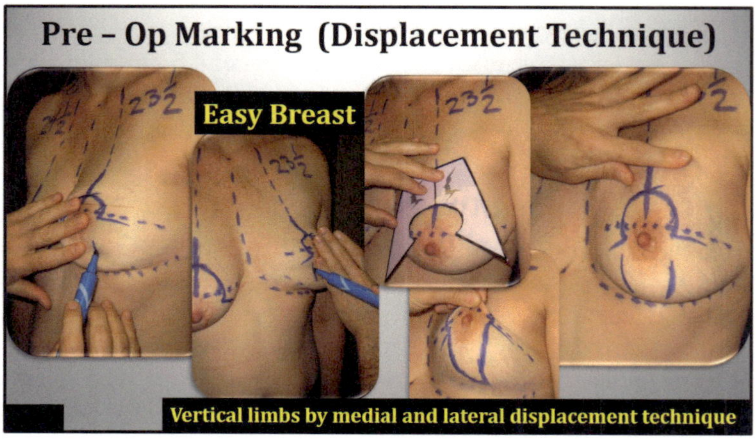

Figure 9.
Marking for a simultaneous lift/augmentation is always performed with the patients standing and arms to the side. As shown for limited ptosis case, the vertical mastopexy marks are along the nature breast axis after lateral and medial displacement of the parenchyma. The base of the vertical must stop 1–2 cm above the IMF to prevent scarring below the fold after closure.

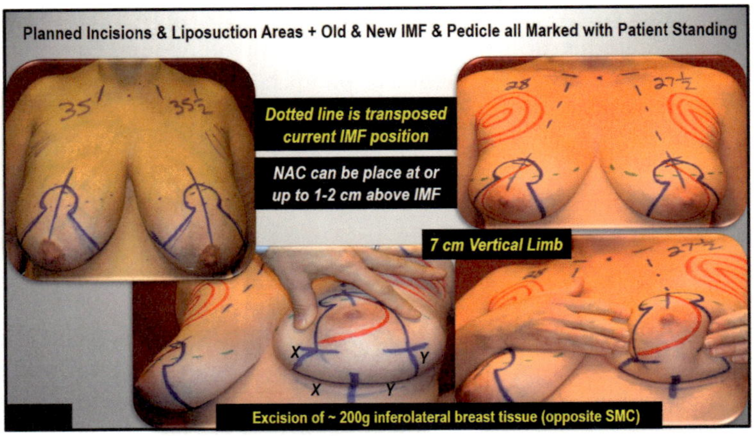

Figure 10.
Marking a planned inverted T incision for a lift/augmentation on a larger breast is similar to marking a vertical mastopexy until vertical limbs are complete. Next, the horizontal incision is typically placed approximately 1 cm above the planned IMF and horizontal limbs kept as short as possible to match the residual skin on each side of the breast axis line as shown (X, Y).

distance to a greater degree (**Figure 10**). When marking the vertical and horizontal limbs of the pattern, it is advisable to err on the side of more conservative resection, given that volume will be added by the implant. Some flexibility in the surgery is added by using implant sizers during the procedure and having multiple implant sizes available intraoperatively. Occasionally, it may be beneficial to use either a larger or smaller implant than initially planned for.

8.2 Anesthesia

General anesthesia is required when performing this procedure given the amount of muscle manipulation. However, tumescent local anesthesia can facilitate easier dissection and resection while minimizing the depth of general anesthesia required. This will decrease postoperative pain requirements and risk of nausea and vomiting, both of which can complicate the early postoperative period. A modified Klein solution (0.5% lidocaine with 1:500,000 epinephrine) is injected into the planned incisions, subpectorally and most importantly into the dermis in the areas of planned de-epithelialization. This is typically done preoperatively in the OR with the patient asleep after a quick prep with alcohol or 4% chlorhexidine. Once administered the patient is reprepped and draped in standard fashion.

8.3 Technique

The surgery is initiated by placing an areolar imprint with an appropriately sized areolar marker centered over the nipple itself. Then, partial thickness incisions are made, followed by de-epithelialization within the planned incisions. Caution is a must so not to undermine the new NAC. While removal of excess fat and gland helps improve shape and longevity, care must be used to leave adequate tissue below the NAC (central pedicle) as well as adequate tissue below each vertical limb. This is followed by development of the pedicle, and en bloc resection of excess or ptotic glandular tissue (**Figure 11**). Typically resecting portions of the inferior, lateral and superolateral area of the keyhole are common for the SMC pedicle. More is removed from the inferior glandular tissues versus less resection superiorly. However sufficient tissue must be removed from the keyhole area to allow inset of the NAC and pedicle without compression or congestion. The inferior excision is completed

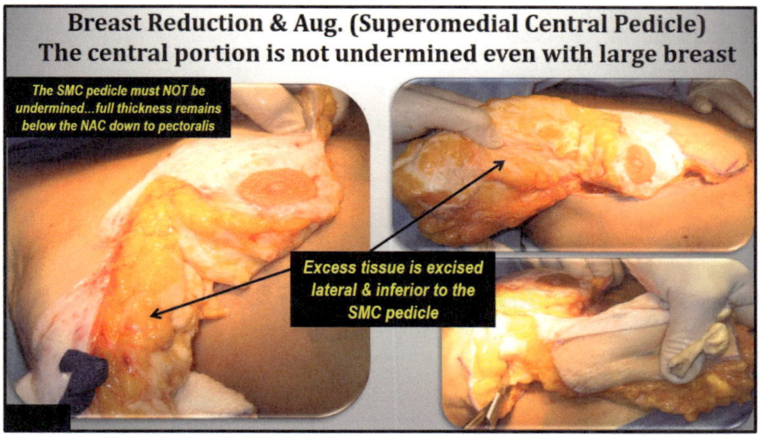

Figure 11.
Excision of redundant skin as well as fat and parenchyma is critical for long term maintenance of the lift. But, as shown, care must be used to not remove too much tissue below the NAC and avoid thinning the flaps below the vertical limbs.

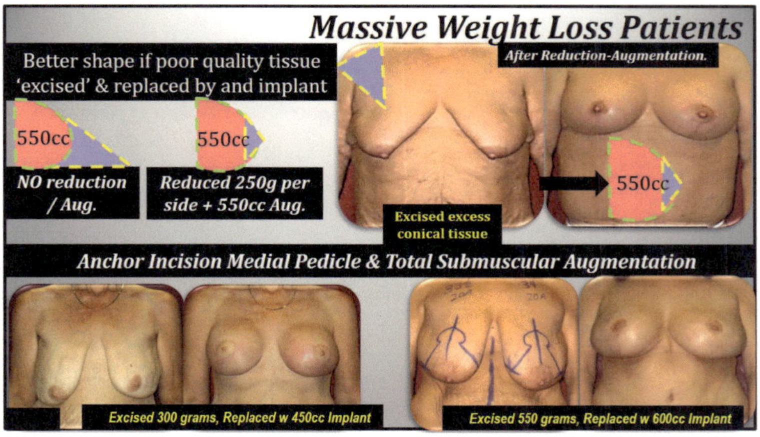

Figure 12.
Three separate patients are shown who lost over 100 lbs. by gastric bypass prior to having simultaneous mastopexy and augmentation. The key for this subset of patients is to remove as much of the excess poor quality mammary tissue and fat as well as skin. This is especially helpful when the breast shape is constricted or conical.

down to the level of the pectoral fascia, but without insult or injury. Excision of tissue is especially important in massive weight loss patients whose residual excess tissue will sag later if not removed (**Figure 12**). Excising as much as possible safely on this subset of patients and allowing a larger implant will produce better longevity and appearance compared to excising little tissue and use of a smaller implant (**Figure 13**). After excision, attention is taken to expose only the inferolateral aspect of the pectoral border for a few centimeters medially. This will allow myotomy paralleling the fibers of the pectoralis major into the postpectoral space while not injuring the central deep component of the glandular pedicle. Once in the postpectoral space, circumferential blunt dissection is initiated with a finger. Inferolaterally, using a sweeping maneuver with the forefinger it is typically easy to lift fibers of the anterior serratus and external oblique muscles (**Figure 14**). Occasionally it may be necessary to utilize limited cutting cautery to aid in pocket development. Once the total submuscular pocket is developed, a lighted retractor will aid in minor sub

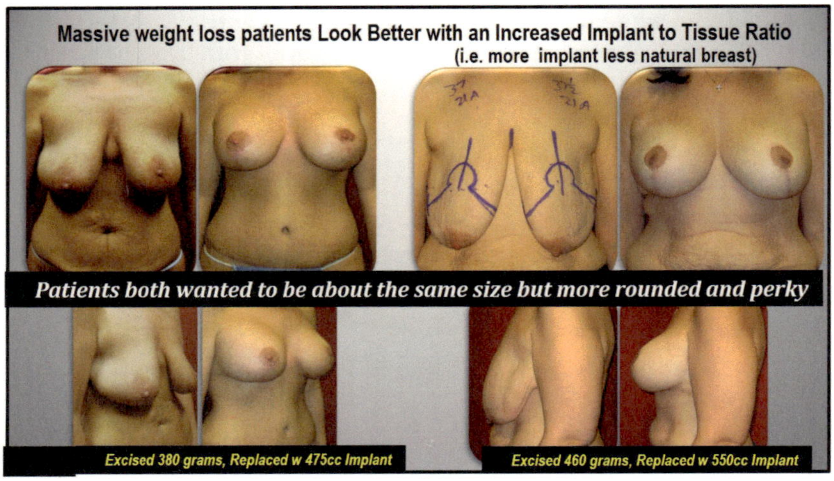

Figure 13.
Massive weight loss patients who desire to be the "same size" but "round and perky" typically will not be happy with a mastopexy alone because of the poor quality of residual tissue. Reduction and augmentation is required as shown to obtain the results most patients will find pleasing.

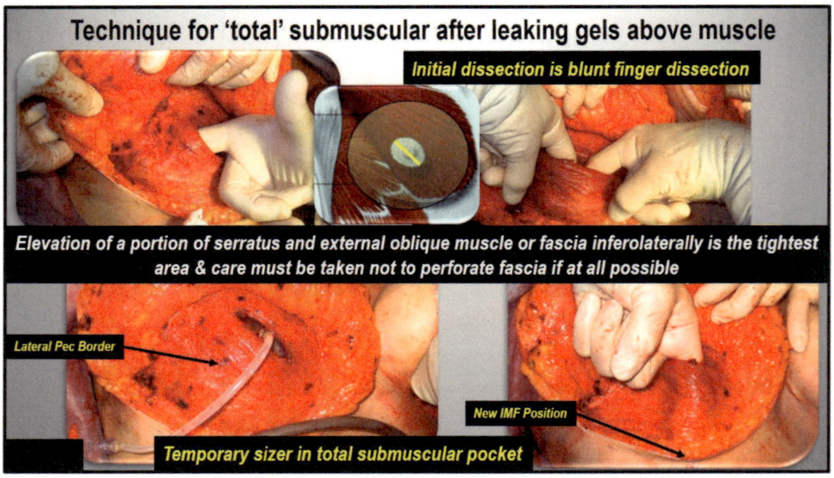

Figure 14.
Elevation of a "total" submuscular coverage pocket is shown during initial finger sweeping. Slow, cautious elevation inferomedially prevents perforation of the flap that is thinner in that location. Lighted retractors are used past initial finger dissection for residual elevation as required and hemostasis.

muscular release if needed for inferior pole expansion and with hemostasis within the pocket. Hemostasis must be performed and verified at multiple points throughout the surgery. After verifying the pedicle and NAC transpose easily into position, the superior trifurcation is closed at the deep dermal level and the NAC pexied into position. Preventing excessive tension at this point greatly improves final scar formation (**Figure 15**). Total submuscular coverage also takes some pressure off the incision line and aids in longevity (**Figure 16**). A sizer can then be placed into the sub muscular pocket and inflated to the desired size. This maneuver can help with assessing implant pocket dimensions and expected tension on the NAC and superior trifurcation closure. The sizer can then be replaced with the corresponding implant and the remaining incisions can then be closed in standard layered fashion with care to carefully align the skin edges and evenly distribute pleating throughout the mastopexy incisions. Glandular pillars may be reapproximated gently with 1–2 resorbable

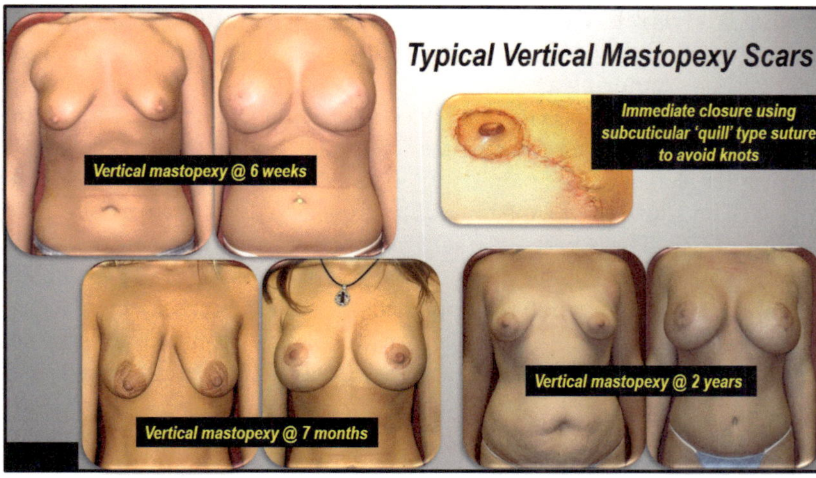

Figure 15.
The vertical limb of the mastopexy greatly improves the scar appearance around the areolas by decreasing radially pressure away from the center. As the patient examples demonstrate, the vertical incision is often required to decrease the diameter of the NAC or at least prevent widening that can often be seen from a donut mastopexy.

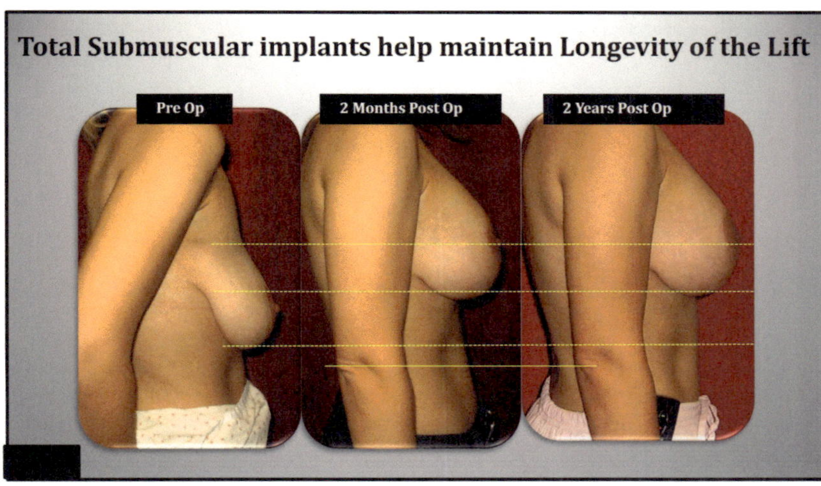

Figure 16.
Demonstration of the longevity benefits from excision of excess glandular tissue as well as total submuscular coverage of the implant as shown. Recurrent ptosis is it occurs is typically from patient weight gain and enlargement of tissue above the implant.

sutures as required to improve shape and projection. Over plication must be avoided. Occasionally, it may be beneficial to perform minor liposuction to the lateral breast if excess fat or fullness at the lateral pole of the incision is present.

9. Revision mastopexy/augmentation

Revision mastopexy/augmentation surgery can be quite difficult but also very rewarding and is a necessary component for anyone offering these procedures. The acknowledgment of an undetermined blood supply and the potential for NAC ischemia is paramount when considering revision surgery. Although prior operative reports may be beneficial, they can be unreliable as to the actual pedicle utilized and great caution must be used. Avoidance of wide excision patterns or significant undermining is advisable. Occasionally multiple pedicles can be combined in some situations to help limit ischemia when the prior pedicle use is unknown (**Figure 17**). Foremost, patients requiring a second mastopexy with or without implant replacement should be informed and educated about potential loss of skin and/or the NAC. Some revision cases may require staging, particularly if they have large subglandular implants, due to the inability to depend on accessory central blood supply to the nipple. The addition of capsular contracture and need for capsulectomy adds even more risk. These patients likely require explantation and capsulectomy first followed by revision mastopexy/augmentation secondarily. When choosing to perform a simultaneous revision mastopexy augmentation and pocket exchange the surgeon must be extra diligent to limit any maneuver that compromises vascularity more than absolutely required (**Figure 18**). The pectoral artery branches have

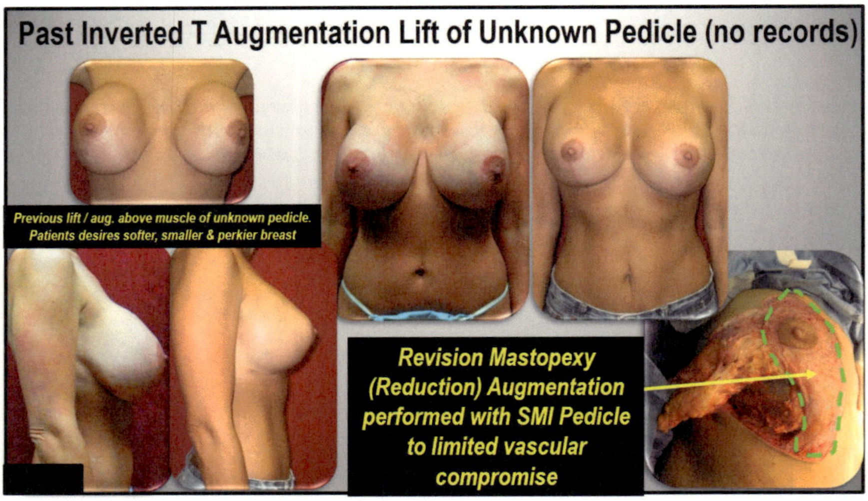

Figure 17.
Patients who have had previous mastopexy & augmentation of an unknown pedicle type present potentially more risk. When possible, using limited dissection and a combined pedicle such as the superomedial-inferior (SMI) shown can avoid unwanted disruption of already decreased vascularity to the NAC.

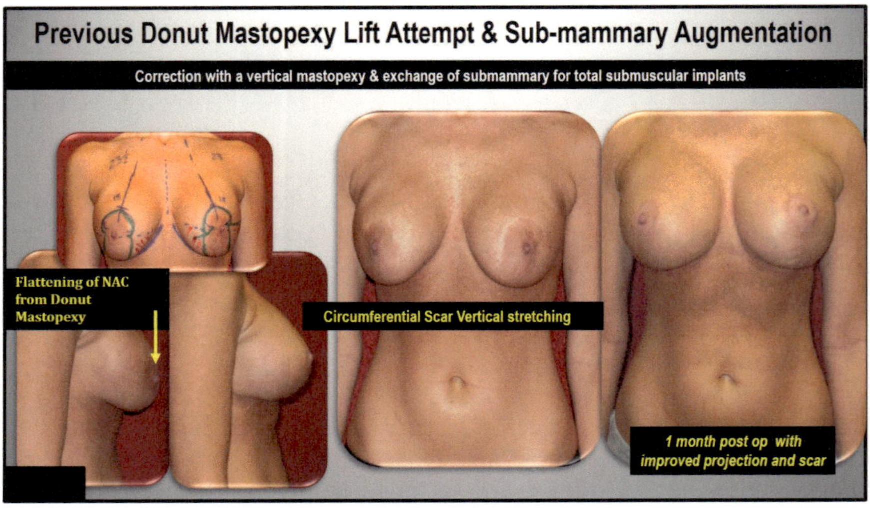

Figure 18.
The patient shown has the classic problem from a circumferential mastopexy that stretched vertically and residual ptosis. She was corrected by complete capsulectomies, new total submuscular implants and revision vertical mastopexy.

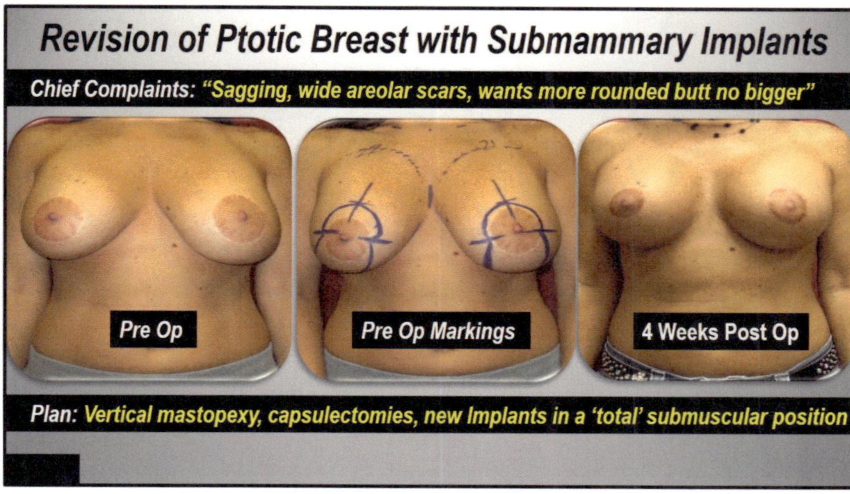

Figure 19.
Revision on a patient who had a circumferential mastopexy and the more common widening pattern of scar formation. The patient wanted smaller areola with better scars, perkier breast and slightly smaller size breast than before.

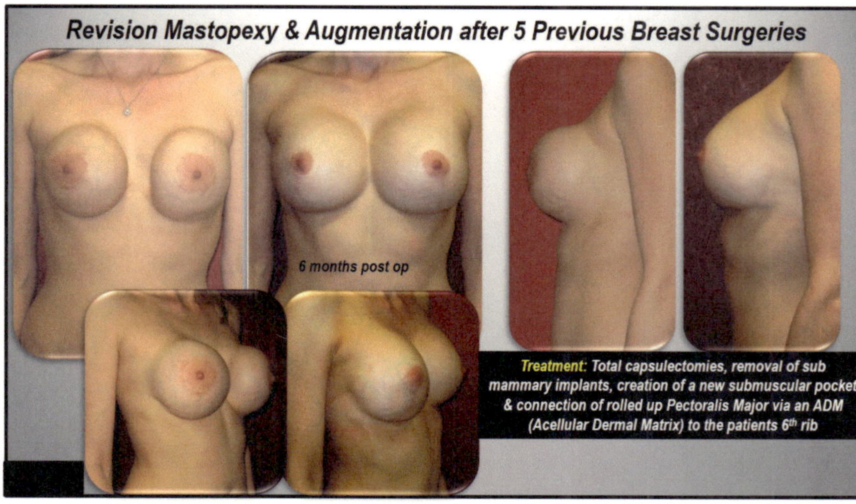

Figure 20.
The figure demonstrates revision on a patient with multiple past surgeries of various types and chronic history of capsular contracture. Damage to the residual muscle necessitates the use of an acellular dermal matrix to connect the residual lateral pectoralis border to the new IMF.

already been severed from the past Submammary augmentation removing the normal central pedicle portion of vascularity.

Unsatisfactory scarring is typically the most required revision and fortunately is often fairly straightforward. The opposing forces of mastopexy skin excision and augmenting breast volume may lead to widened and unsatisfactory scars on occasion. This is usually remedied with standard scar revision techniques and has a high rate of success with a careful tension free closure. NAC irregularity or asymmetry can be seen and is typically improved best by adding a vertical incision to reduce tension around the NAC. Of particular note is the tendency for isolated periareolar lifts to widen with time, independent of suture type used and especially when combined with augmentation (**Figure 19**). The proper correction of this relies on the addition of a small vertical

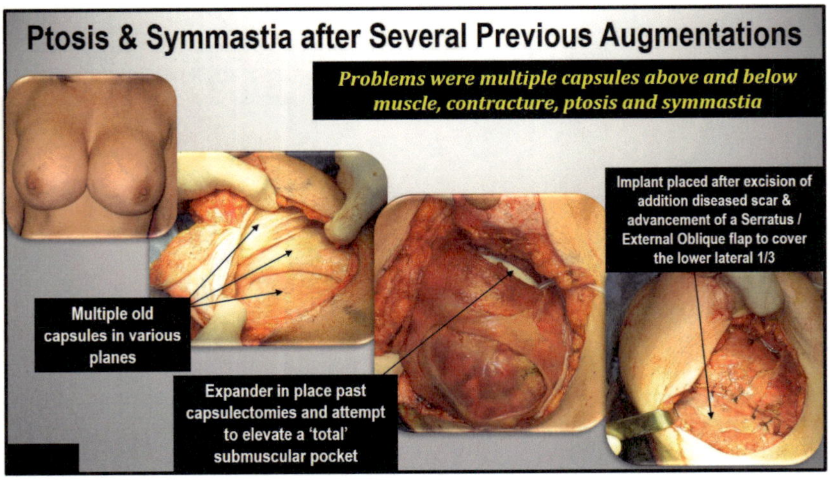

Figure 21.
Damage to the residual muscle shown was corrected by excising the old capsules from multiple surgeries and developing an inferolateral submuscular flap to elevate the serratus and external oblique as shown. Recruited muscle and fascia was used in place of an ADM.

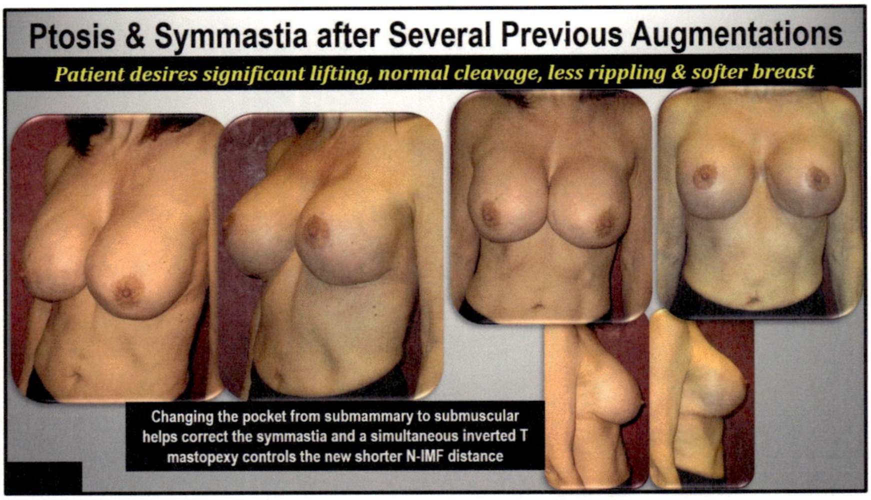

Figure 22.
Simultaneous correction of ptosis and symmastia was performed using an inverted T mastopexy because of the extent of excess skin and new pocket creation to correct the symmastia.

component with periareolar revision. This will take tension off the new areolar diameter and return a more conical appliance to the breast that is often flattened with Benelli-type lifts.

Implant malposition is a common complication with augmentation alone and is certainly encountered with post mastopexy/augmentation. The most common malposition is inferiorly and laterally. Standard pocket modification procedures are similarly beneficial as they are post augmentation alone. However, soft tissue reinforcement may be required as some patients will have less than desired intrinsic tissue integrity. Acellular dermis and bio-resorbable silk derived scaffolds are the mainstays of tissue reinforcement in reconstructive cases and have been used with success in the revision of cosmetic breast cases (**Figure 20**) [3]. This is particularly true when capsular contracture exists and multiple surgeries in the past have taken place. Occasional localized adjacent muscle flaps can be used to cover the gaps and gain better implant coverage (**Figure 21**). Revision of symmastia if found simultaneously with ptosis issues requires either staging, new pocket development, or ADM usage (**Figure 22**).

10. Complications

As with even simple breast surgery, there is a notable complication rate. Consistently, studies have shown 15–25% reoperation rates post primary augmentation, and clinical experience shows that this rate is consistent when augmentation is combined with mastopexy [10]. Interestingly, these studies have shown the complication rates to not be exponential or even additive when combined surgery is performed versus a two stage approach [11, 12]. This is likely explained by the occasional patient specific intrinsic difficulties associated with either mastopexy and augmentation alone along with more careful patient selection when combining procedures. And fortunately, significant complications like implant extrusion, infection and nipple necrosis are very uncommon. Should nipple ischemia be noted intraoperatively, several maneuvers may reverse the impending danger. Evacuation of periareolar hematoma and strict hemostasis is the simplest step, otherwise nitroglycerin paste or spray immediately postoperatively to the NAC for minor ischemia is beneficial by improving venous congestion. However, should the ischemia be more profound, early removal of sutures and/or the implant will likely improve blood supply and venous drainage. Lastly, consideration of hyperbaric therapy in the early postoperative period, although cumbersome and not well defined in the literature, has shown evidence of dramatic reversal in impending necrosis [13]. Fortunately, the most significant reasons for reoperation are typically unfavorable scarring, capsular contracture, hematoma and implant malposition [14]. Excising entire capsules because of capsular contracture increases risk of hematoma especially when combined with ptosis correction (**Figure 23**). These are managed in a similar manner for either augmentation or mastopexy alone and methods to minimize these complications and the need for subsequent revisions are not very different than for either mastopexy or augmentation alone. For instance, the authors do not perform mastopexy surgery on current smokers for well-defined reasons, and of course this

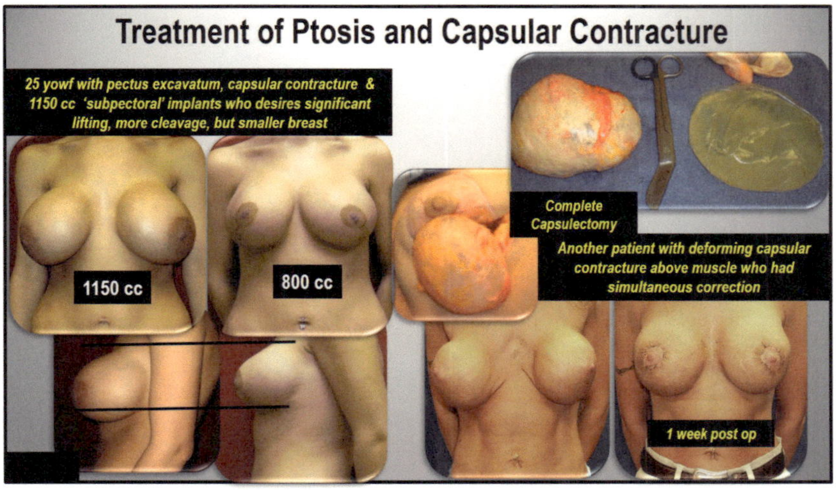

Figure 23.
Simultaneous correction of ptosis and capsular contracture adds to an already high revision rate and complication rate of simultaneous mastopexy/augmentation. The patients shown are even higher risk because of thin tissue and large implant size.

includes candidates for simultaneous surgery as well. As previously mentioned, a more conservative methodology for implant size selection is recommended in combined surgery in order to minimize wound tension and ischemic stress on the NAC. Otherwise, simultaneous mastopexy and augmentation is planned with a similar risk stratification to other cosmetic breast procedures, albeit with more regard for the rarer more devastating complications discussed above [15].

11. Summary

Simultaneous mastopexy and augmentation is challenging, but also highly rewarding and well accepted by informed patients. A clear understanding of not only the individual procedures, but the added variables involved when combining these techniques will greatly aid the surgeon in obtaining safe and predictable results while keeping the vast majority of complications relatively minor.

Author details

Angelo Cuzalina[1*] and Landon McLain[2]

1 Tulsa Surgical Arts, USA

2 McLain Surgical Arts, Huntsville, USA

*Address all correspondence to: angelo@tulsasurgicalarts.com

References

[1] Netter FH. Atlas of Human Anatomy. 2nd ed. Philadelphia: PA, Novartis; 1997. p. 525

[2] Hauben DJ, Adler N, Silfen R, Regev D. Breast-areola-nipple proportion. Annals of Plastic Surgery. 2003;**50**(5):510-513

[3] Spear SL, Willey SC, Robb GL, Hammond DC, Nahabedian MY. Surgery of the Breast: Principles and Art. 2nd ed. Philadelphia: Lippincott Williams and Williams; 2006. p. 1517

[4] Nahai F. The Art of Aesthetic Surgery: Principles and Techniques. 2nd ed. St. Louis: MO, Quality Medical Publishing; 2011. p. 3187

[5] Hall-Findlay EJ, Spear SL, Davison SP. New trends in reduction and mastopexy vertical breast reduction. Seminars in Plastic Surgery. 2004;**18**(3):211-224

[6] Brown RH, Siy R, Khan K, Izaddoost S. The superomedial pedicle wise-pattern breast reduction: Reproducible, reliable, and resilient. Seminars in Plastic Surgery. 2015;**29**(2):94-101

[7] Nahabedian MY, McGibbon BM, Manson PN. Medial pedicle reduction mammaplasty for severe mammary hypertrophy. Plastic and Reconstructive Surgery. Philadelphia: PA; 2000;**105**(3):896-904

[8] Aston SJ, Steinbrach DS, Walden JL. Aesthetic Plastic Surgery. Saunders Elsevier; 2009. p. 946

[9] Henriksen TF, Fryzek JP, Holmich LR, et al. Surgical intervention and capsular contracture after breast augmentation: A prospective study of risk factors. Annals of Plastic Surgery. 2005;**54**:343-351

[10] Gutowski KA, Mesna GT, Cunningham BL. Saline-filled breast implants: A plastic surgery educational foundation multicenter outcomes study. Plastic and Reconstructive Surgery. 1997;**100**:1019-1027

[11] Adams WP Jr. Discussion: Simultaneous augmentation mastopexy a retrospective 5-year review of 332 consecutive cases. Plastic and Reconstructive Surgery. 2013;**131**(1):157-158

[12] Stevens WG, Macias LH, Spring M, Stoker DA, Chacón CO, Eberlin SA. One-stage augmentation mastopexy: A review of 1192 simultaneous breast augmentation and mastopexy procedures in 615 consecutive patients. Aesthetic Surgery Journal. 2014;**34**(5):723-732

[13] Copeland-Halperin LR, Bruce SB, Mesbahi AN. Hyperbaric oxygen following bilateral skin-sparing mastectomies: A case report. Plastic and Reconstructive Surgery. Global Open. 2016;**4**(4):e680

[14] Stevens WG, Nahabedian MY, Calobrace MB, et al. Risk factor analysis for capsular contracture: A 5-year Sientra study analysis using round, smooth, and textured implants for breast augmentation. Plastic and Reconstructive Surgery. 2013;**132**:1115-1123

[15] Calobrace MB, Herdt DRBS, Cothron KJ. Simultaneous augmentation/mastopexy: A retrospective 5-year review of 332 consecutive cases. Plastic and Reconstructive Surgery. 2013;**131**(1):145-156

Section 2

Abdominal and Gluteal Contouring

Chapter 3

Helium Plasma-Driven Radiofrequency in Body Contouring

Diane Irvine Duncan

Abstract

Consumer demand for a minimally invasive alternative to dermolipectomy-based excisional procedures has been driven by interest in risk reduction, reduced scarring in the treatment region, and significant lessening of recovery time. While minimally invasive liposuction is a common approach, limitations can include residual skin laxity and irregular skin contour. The current literature suggests that radio frequency energy is superior in achieving non-excisional soft tissue and skin shrinkage without surgical skin resection. Monopolar and bipolar radiofrequency-based devices have been available for 10 years. Recently, a plasma-driven radiofrequency device, Renuvion, was introduced and FDA cleared for soft tissue coagulation. The device uses a pressurized helium tank to drive radiofrequency energy into a hollow cannula. As measured skin temperature rarely exceeds 38°C, the safety profile of the device is optimized. The use of helium-driven plasma energy is a new and promising resource for achieving non-excisional soft tissue and skin tightening. Because the device rapidly heats subcutaneous collagen, strong immediate contraction is generated within fractions of a second. This treatment is followed by very visible improvement at the 24 hour post-op mark. Results can continue to improve over a year, as infiltration of new collagen within the adipose stroma occurs.

Keywords: skin tightening, radiofrequency, impedance based, minimally invasive, helium plasma

1. Introduction

For decades, the ability to reshape the human body was limited to dermolipectomy-based excisional procedures with long scars. Consumer demand for a minimally invasive alternative has been driven by interest in risk reduction, reduced scarring in the treatment region, and significant lessening of recovery time so that patients can return to work or regular activity within a short time span. Liposuction appeared to be the golden solution for many. While this minimally invasive procedure is a common approach, limitations can include residual skin laxity, an irregular skin contour, and little improvement in regions that were pendulous prior to the procedure. Subcutaneous tone is generally not improved with traditional suction-assisted lipectomy (SAL). Goals other than fat reduction include significant skin and soft tissue contraction in a smooth and even manner. While ultrasound and laser-assisted lipoplasty have been recommended for this purpose following liposuction, consistent outcomes have not been able to be achieved. The current literature suggests that radiofrequency (RF) energy is superior in achieving non-excisional soft tissue and skin shrinkage without surgical skin resection. By targeting the subcutaneous collagen matrix instead of just the skin, practitioners of body contouring are able to achieve up to 36% measured skin surface area contraction at 1 year following treatment with RF-assisted liposuction. While monopolar and bipolar radiofrequency-based devices for this purpose have been available for 10 years, only recently has a plasma-driven radiofrequency device been in introduced. The Renuvion device is FDA cleared for the purpose of soft tissue coagulation. The device is a modification of a standard Bovie electrocautery unit. The new configuration has a pressurized helium tank attached to the energy delivery system, so that helium plasma-driven energy is emitted from a hollow cannula when the device is activated. The handpiece is moved in the subdermal plane in a manner similar to that of a liposuction cannula. Emitted energy is fractional. Small fragments of stromal collagen are heated very quickly to 85°C, causing a reduction in fiber length of 40–50%.

Because the measured skin temperature rarely exceeds 38°C, the safety profile of the device is optimized. Soft tissue treatment is usually performed following liposuction, but it can also be used in the subcutaneous plane without liposuction when skin contraction alone is desired. The use of the device for these purposes is considered off label.

2. History of suction-assisted lipectomy (SAL)

Patient and physician interest in limiting incisions and complications led to the development of liposuction in the late 1970s [1]. While Illouz [2] has commonly been given credit for coming up with liposuction as a new procedure, other surgeons before him used a combination of sharp cannulas without tumescent fluid to remove fat. German surgeons Schrudde, Meyer, and Kesselring performed liposuction in the early to the mid-1970s in such a manner [3]. Blood loss was significant, and clinical outcomes were not ideal.

The Fischers, a father and son team, developed a blunt liposuction cannula in the mid-1970s [4].

They treated only the thigh area. Frenchmen Illouz and Fournier spread the technique to other body regions and to other esthetic surgeons [5]. During the late 1970s, they began combining injection of intravenous fluid and hyaluronidase for the purpose of improving the ease of dissection. The term they used was "wet technique." Klein [6] is credited with the concept of tumescent fluid, which differs from the French wet technique by adding both epinephrine (to reduce intraoperative blood loss) and lidocaine (for pain reduction during the procedure, so that it could be performed while the patient was awake). Sodium bicarbonate was added to the injectable fluid in order to reduce burning on injection when general anesthesia was not used. The safety of infusing large volumes of this solution was documented in studies performed by the dermatologic surgery contingent, who focused on lidocaine toxicity [7]. The complication rate with liposuction was significant though [8], and the ASAPS recommended limiting large volumes of infusion and lipoaspirate over 5 L to the hospital setting [9].

Liposuction rapidly gained popularity but did not replace dermolipectomy, as limited skin surface area contraction was noted with SAL alone [10]. The development of energy-assisted liposuction was rapid and included ultrasound, laser, power, water-jet, shock wave, and radiofrequency-assisted liposuction [11–16].

While many new devices have been utilized during the past 20 years, few have attained the simultaneous goal of significant and esthetically acceptable skin contraction in the treatment region.

For decades, practitioners and patients alike have been focused on treating "skin laxity" without considering the true cause of the problem. Recent publications [17] show that the adipose/stromal framework of the skin may be a better treatment target. Rubin noted [18] that skin follows the substructure. If the scaffold or framework that the skin rests upon is weak or ptotic, the skin will follow, as it has no ability to hold a fixed shape on its own. If a practitioner chooses a device or treatment that does not target the framework, also known as the fibroseptal network (FSN), the goal of improving a pendulous structure will not be met without an excisional approach.

How does the skin become lax? Facial aging studies show that the average person loses 235 cc of bony mass during a lifetime [19]. Certainly, there is associated muscle and fat atrophy with aging [20, 21]. While fat loss in the face and neck is a normal part of the aging process, these factors do not explain the loss of soft tissue tone. Serial scanning electron micrographs were taken from volunteers of various ages and similar skin types [22]. These show that with age, weight gain and loss, and genetic predilection, the stromal portion of the adipose framework for the overlying skin becomes weak, due to loss of the fibrocollagenous matrix and involution of the vascular network.

While mechanical stimulation of the FSN with liposuction can create an 8% skin surface area contraction at 1 year posttreatment [23], the firm tone and defined shape of youthful body contours are not re-established. A thermal regenerative solution for this dilemma has been the focus of my energy-based device studies over the last decade.

3. History of energy-based devices

Ultrasound-assisted liposuction (UAL) was introduced by Zocchi in 1990 [24]. Reports of complications including seroma, burns, and contour irregularities caused a loss of popularity of this particular device. A current ultrasound-based device, Vaser, is still in regular use but is not targeted toward causing skin contraction. Power-assisted liposuction (PAL) is used by many practitioners who like the vibratory nature of the handpiece for treatment of fibrous areas and in secondary cases. Water-jet-assisted liposuction is excellent for fat grafting harvest, but does not improve the overall liposuction outcome. Laser-assisted liposuction (LAL) was shown to create a 13–17% skin surface area reduction at 3–6 months post-op [12]. Lack of a long-term outcome has led to a loss in popularity of this device. Radiofrequency-based tissue tightening has increased in popularity as longer-term improvement has been shown [23]. A bipolar device with indwelling liposuction capability was introduced in 2008 (Invasix) [16], and a monopolar device was cleared for soft tissue coagulation in 2012 (Thermi) [25]. This device utilized a subcutaneous cannula with an internal temperature probe. In 2012, a new version of the bipolar device (InMode) was introduced that contained both internal and external temperature monitors. A 50% improvement in upper arm pendulosity and a 36% skin surface area reduction at 1 year were seen with this device [26]. In 2016, the J-Plasma device (Bovie Medical) was introduced for the purpose of subdermal coagulation. The device was originally developed as a general surgical/gyn/urological laparoscopic cautery device. In esthetic cases, the cannula with blade retracted has been used in the subcutaneous plane for the purpose of collagen coagulation.

4. Mechanical effects of liposuction

Traditional SAL removes fat. However, the procedure is also a mechanical, nonthermal FSN stimulant. If simple fat reduction in a young patient with no soft tissue laxity is the goal, then fat removal and mechanical stimulation of the soft tissue will cause some reduction of the distended skin and soft tissue mass. Nonthermal trauma to the tissue induces an inflammatory response, which as we know causes inosculation of new blood vessels, generation of fibroblasts, and formation of new collagen or scar tissue within the treated space. Chemokines, cytokines, and growth factors all influence tissue response to mechanical injury [27]. Skin contraction with SAL measures about 10% at 6–8 weeks posttreatment [23] and then relaxes to a measured 8% skin surface area contraction at 1 year.

Practitioners such as specialists like Gasparoni and Toledo used superficial liposuction to optimize skin shrinkage [28]. However, reports of complications resulting from treatment by other surgeons have diminished the popularity of this procedure [29]. Full-thickness skin loss due to aggressive superficial liposuction is still a concern, especially in Central and South America.

5. Thermal effects of heating soft tissue

When heat is added to mechanical stimulation, the soft tissue response changes. Thermal effects of radiofrequency energy can include ablation, coagulation, and collagen contraction [30]. While ablation without adjacent tissue damage is a desired goal in vaporizing tumors or lesions, the esthetic practitioner has more commonly used RF to cauterize blood vessels or to directly shrink soft tissue. Common use of a pencil-type cautery unit includes shrinkage of the SMAS in face lifting or a "popcorn" capsulorrhaphy in breast implant surgery.

A newer concept is that of contraction of collagen fibers, a microeffect of RF energy on the tissue. Genin [31] notes that the native state of triple helical collagen strands change to a transitional state and then become denatured when temperature from the device over time causes the protein to unfold. In a study by Rossman [32], he showed that average collagen fibers measure 290 nm shrank to 101.5 nm when denatured, a contraction of 65%.

The electric properties of tissue are governed by impedance or "resistivity" to energy conductance [33]. When a uniform tissue type is exposed to radiofrequency energy, impedance can be measured using a certain cross section with a measured distance between the electrodes [30]. Blood is highly conductive to RF energy with a slight lowering of impedance between 0 and 6 MHz. Its conductivity coefficient is 0.7 (low impedance), while fat has high impedance with a conductivity coefficient of 0.03. The value of adding tumescent fluid to fat is illustrated by contrasting the impedance of dry and wet skin. Dry skin conducts RF energy at a 0.03 coefficient—the same as fat, while wet skin has a 0.25 coefficient.

If tissue is heating slightly—elevating the temperature from 37°C to 44°C, the metabolic process quickens [34]. At 45°C, there is a structural change in the collagen helix which leads to hyperthermic cell death. At 60–80°C, collagen proteins denature and unfold. At 90°C, tissues become dessicated, and at 100°C, they become thermally ablated.

In treating patients, factors to consider include the "permittivity" of the tissue to heat, and the temperature achieved in the treatment region. These two factors, as well as duration of energy exposure, directly influence clinical outcome. The vascular perfusion to the area is another very important consideration. This can be compromised in patients who have had previous procedures in the treatment zone. The frequency and type of energy source will also affect tissue response.

6. Radiofrequency energy in esthetic procedures

Energy has been applied in some form to tissue since the beginning of recorded history. The practice of applying heat to tissue through the use of cauters was used for thousands of years as an invaluable method of controlling hemorrhage. Continuous improvement of methods for utilizing the beneficial effects of heat on tissue eventually led to the development of the basic concepts of electrosurgery we know today. In October of 1926, Dr. Harvey Cushing used an electrosurgical unit developed by Dr. William T. Bovie to successfully remove a highly vascularized brain tumor from a patient after previous failed attempts. Today, electrosurgical instruments are used in the majority of surgical procedures performed worldwide [35].

Radiofrequency-based devices for skin rejuvenation became popular in the early 1990s, as a noninvasive device (Thermage) was used to improve tissue tone and texture. Other devices rapidly followed and utilized monopolar, bipolar, and multipolar configurations to treat the skin surface. While the Bovie cautery device has been used for decades in the subcutaneous plane, an open approach was needed. The first subdermal device to be used in a minimally invasive manner was the BodyTite device, which in 2008 had an accompanying liposuction cannula. The monopolar Thermi device utilizes a 10- or 15-cm slender monopolar cannula in a subdermal manner to heat soft tissue at the level of the fibroseptal network. These devices are characterized as "bulk heating" devices and create a radiant pattern of tissue heating from the probe tip outward.

7. Characteristics of bulk heating devices

Traditional subcutaneous monopolar and bipolar radiofrequency devices utilize a small cannula that is placed underneath the skin to heat the adipose tissue. They are called bulk heaters because the thermal energy generated from the tip of the device heats the adjacent tissue from the point of emanation. The surrounding tissue becomes warm gradually in a radiant distribution. Monopolar RF has only a single source of subcutaneous energy, and heat must accumulate in the tissue from this small point. A grounding pad is needed to safely treat the patient (**Figure 1**). Bipolar devices maintain a zone of energy between two sources, in this case, one internal and the other external (**Figure 2**). If the external treatment head is small, it will take a while for the tissue between the two emitters to heat up. Broader external heads create wider fields of heated tissue and are more time efficient. Energy output also influences the speed of tissue heating. Tumesced tissue increases the permittivity of the adipose layer toward heat. If liposuction is indicated, it should be performed prior to energy application. Then, tissue heating is optimized, as the heat-resistant adipose shield will have been removed from the collagen bands of the fibroseptal network, which have lower impedance. Advantages of these device types include ease of use, a known performance history, and many experienced users. Limitations include a long duration of heating if treatment areas are broad. Even with an external sensor such as a FLIR camera or external thermistor, burns and seromas can occur. Clinical endpoints of treatment include warmth, erythema, and a slight tissue reaction when the cannula is moved under the skin. While the internal cannula tip can get to the preset temperature quickly, the surrounding tissue takes time to get warm. Thus, there are "hot spots," which may

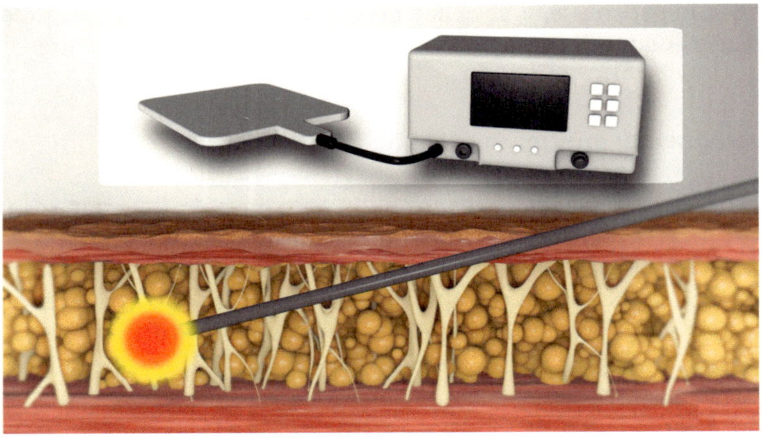

Figure 1.
Monopolar soft tissue coagulation device. The heated tissue radius is small, as the cannula tip is not large. There is a central region that heats to a high temperature, but this rapidly drops down at the periphery. A grounding pad is needed in order to safely treat the patient.

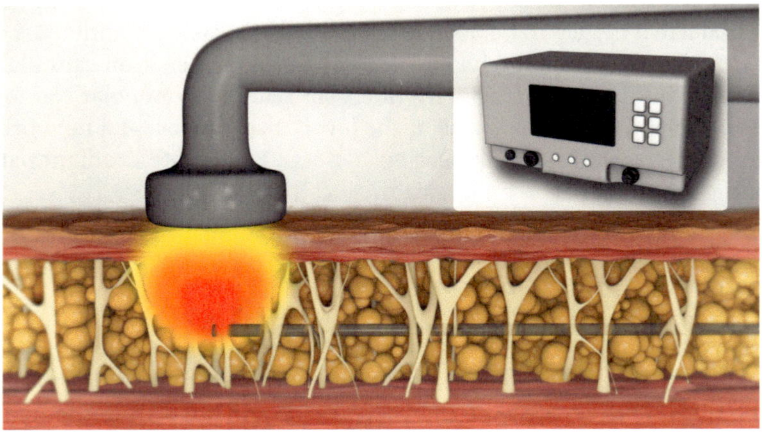

Figure 2.
Bipolar configuration of a radiofrequency-assisted tissue tightening device. There is an internal and external heat sensor. The cannula is deployed in the subcutaneous fat in a manner similar to that of a liposuction cannula.

develop seromas, and areas where heating is not optimized. If the operator continues to heat a region that has already been optimally treated, cauterization of the microvasculature can cause ischemia, resulting in fibrosis or a burn. Knowing the amount of energy used is helpful, but a difficulty with any energy-based device is knowing when you are done. Factors that should reduce the amount of time and energy spent include an area with thin skin, a relatively thin layer of fat (such as the neck, face, and decollete), and any degree of existing fibrosis. FLIR studies show that when used in a primary case in the fibrous bra roll region, a bipolar device generated a skin temperature of 45°C for several minutes, even after the device was removed (**Figure 3**), despite the preset skin cutoff temperature being 38°C. A key to success when using these devices is to consider decreasing treatment time and measuring the skin temperature with FLIR in regions that have been previously treated and have some scar tissue and compromised blood supply. In fibrous areas, the physical nature of bulk heating can create a heat sink, due to the slow dispersion of heat. Compromised blood supply due to scarring or physical containment of heat

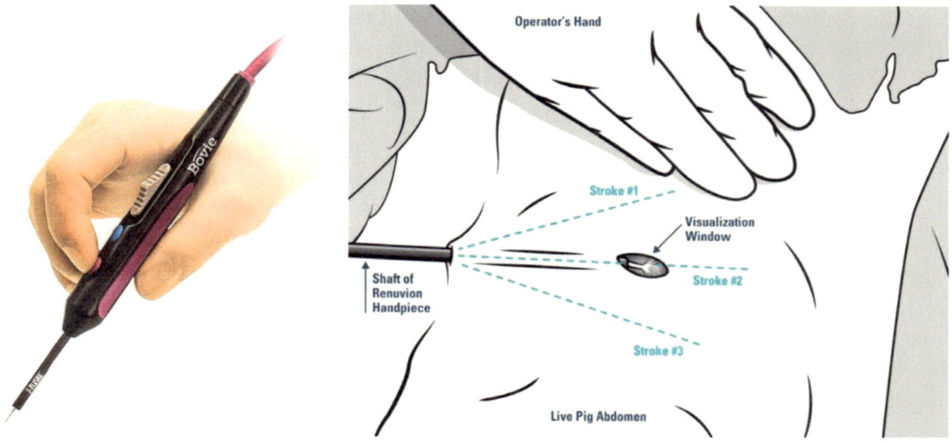

Figure 3.
Illustration of methods used in tissue temperature study.

is a region with fibrous fat which is a relative contraindication to the use of a subcutaneous bulk heating device.

8. Characteristics of the helium plasma-driven device

Bovie Medical Corporation's Renuvion® (formerly branded as J-Plasma®) helium-based plasma technology has FDA clearance for the cutting, coagulation, and ablation of soft tissue. The Renuvion® system consists of an electrosurgical generator unit, a handpiece, and a supply of helium gas. RF energy is delivered to the handpiece by the generator and used to energize an electrode. When helium gas is passed over the energized electrode, a helium plasma is generated which allows heat to be applied to the tissue in two different and distinct ways. First, heat is generated by the actual production of the plasma beam itself through the ionization and rapid neutralization of the helium atoms. Second, since plasmas are very good electrical conductors, a portion of the RF energy used to energize the electrode and generate the plasma passes from the electrode to the patient and heats tissue by passing current through the resistance of the tissue, a process known as Joule heating. These two sources of tissue heating give the Renuvion® device some unique advantages during use as a surgical tool for the coagulation of subcutaneous soft tissue for the purpose of soft tissue contraction.

8.1 Renuvion® instant tissue heating versus bulk tissue heating

Monopolar and bipolar RF devices available for subcutaneous soft tissue coagulation work on the principle of bulk tissue heating. The device is activated until a preset subcutaneous temperature in the range of 65–70°C is achieved and maintained. The tissue being treated must be maintained at that temperature for greater than 120 s for maximal contraction to occur. Although these devices have proven effective in achieving soft tissue contraction [36], the process of heating and maintaining that temperature for extended periods can be time-consuming. In devices without an external temperature monitor, the skin surface can become overheated, causing occasional blisters or burns.

A study conducted on a live porcine model to establish the subdermal tissue temperatures produced by the Renuvion® device demonstrated a different philosophy for achieving soft tissue contraction when compared to the RF devices described above. See **Figure 3** for an illustration of the methods used in this porcine study. The study simulated actual clinical conditions as closely as possible including tumescent infiltration and completion of liposuction on the abdomen of the pig. Prior to beginning treatment with the Renuvion® device, an incision was made through the epidermis and dermis into the subdermal plane to serve as a visualization window through which a forward-looking infrared radiometer (FLIR) camera could measure internal tissue temperatures. Multiple treatment passes of the Renuvion® device were then conducted using a matrix of various treatment combinations. For each treatment combination tested, a single treatment pass consisted of three strokes of the device in the subdermal plane (see **Figure 3**). The second treatment stroke was performed so that the tip of the Renuvion® device passed directly underneath the visualization window. This novel testing method allowed the FLIR camera to capture both internal and external tissue temperatures simultaneously. See **Figure 4** for an example of the images captured by the FLIR camera as the device passes under the visualization window.

Typical results from the porcine study are shown in **Figure 5**. It is important to note that the time shown on the X-axis in this graph is reported in milliseconds.

As shown in **Figure 5**, the Renuvion® device heats the tissue to temperatures greater than 85°C for between 0.040 and 0.080 s [17]. Heating the tissue to these temperatures for this period of time is adequate for achieving maximal soft tissue coagulation and contraction. However, unlike with bulk tissue heating, the tissue surrounding the treatment site remains at much cooler temperatures resulting in rapid cooling after the application of the energy through conductive heat transfer. Published studies have shown that the majority of soft tissue contraction induced by subcutaneous energy delivery devices is due to its effect on the fibroseptal network [12, 13]. Because of these unique heating and cooling properties of the Renuvion® technology, immediate soft tissue contraction can be achieved without unnecessarily heating the full thickness of the dermis. Practitioners who became used to the need for monitoring skin temperatures with a FLIR camera will find this is not needed with the Renuvion system.

Figure 6 helps to visualize the differences between the bulk tissue heating of monopolar and bipolar RF devices and the instant tissue heating of the Renuvion® helium plasma device. The narrow difference between subdermal and epidermal temperatures of the monopolar and bipolar devices (top image in **Figure 6**) results

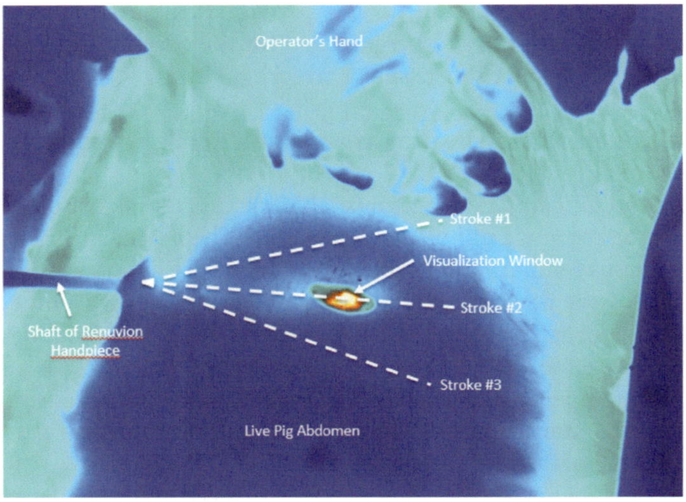

Figure 4.
FLIR camera image.

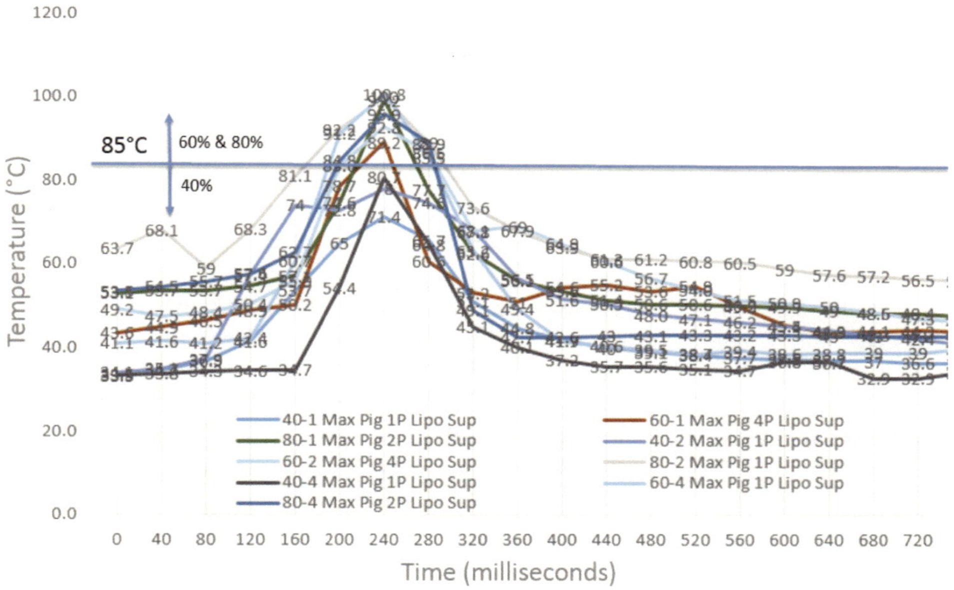

Figure 5.
Temperature vs. time (in ms) for Renuvion treatment [17].

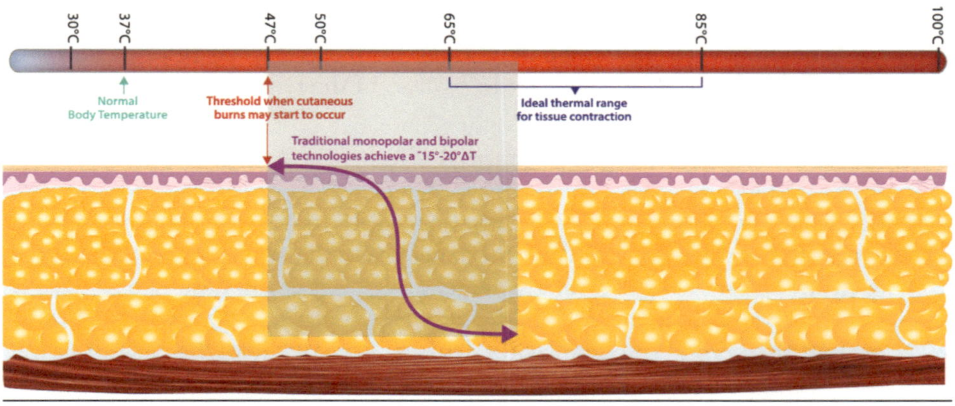

Figure 6.
Differences in epidermal and subdermal temperatures for monopolar and bipolar RF devices (top) and Renuvion® helium plasma device (bottom). Author's note: while a skin temperature of 45°C was noted in the porcine model, the maximum FLIR reading on a human subject's epidermis has been 38°C.

in a delicate balance between achieving the subdermal temperatures needed for soft tissue contraction and maintaining safe epidermal temperatures, resulting in the need for constant internal and external temperature monitoring. A much larger difference between internal and external tissue temperatures for the Renuvion® device (bottom image in **Figure 6**) achieves maximal tissue contraction while maintaining safe skin temperatures without the need for temperature monitoring.

8.2 Renuvion®—360° tissue treatment

It is known that electrical energy takes the path of least resistance. RF energy flows through the conductive plasma beam generated by the Renuvion® system. This conductive plasma beam can be thought of as a flexible wire or electrode that "connects" to the tissue that represents the path of least resistance for the flow of the RF energy. This tissue is typically either that which is in the closest proximity to the tip of the Renuvion® device or the tissue that has the lowest impedance (is the easiest to pass energy through). When used for the coagulation of subcutaneous soft tissue, this means that the energy from the Renuvion® device is not directed or focused in any set direction when activated in the subdermal plane. As the tip of the Renuvion® device is drawn through the subdermal plane, new structures are introduced to the tip of the device, and the path of least resistance is constantly changing. As the energy is constantly finding a new preferred path, the plasma beam quickly alternates direction, seeking out new structures to heat (see **Figure** 7). This allows for 360° tissue treatment without the need for the user to redirect the flow of energy. Since the collagen framework of the FSN is typically the closest tissue to the tip of the Renuvion® device, the vast majority of the energy delivered by the device results in coagulation and contraction of the fibroseptal bands. Maximizing the energy flow to the FSN expedites the soft tissue contraction process.

8.3 Renuvion®—consistent power output

The design of the electrosurgical generator for the Renuvion® plasma device is fundamentally different from that of monopolar and bipolar devices. As shown in **Figure 8**, monopolar and bipolar devices have limited power output in tissues with higher impedance, such as fat. The Renuvion® device was designed to maintain consistent power output over a wide range of impedances. When used for the coagulation of subdermal tissue, the Renuvion® output is not self-limiting and provides unencumbered delivery of power regardless of the tissue impedance.

8.4 Renuvion®—minimal depth of thermal effect

Not all RF energy is created equal. Experienced RF users know that you can achieve very different tissue results at the same power setting by simply changing from an RF waveform designed for cutting to an RF waveform designed for coagulation. The proprietary oscillating waveform of the Renuvion® device has much lower current than typical monopolar RF devices. In most cases, the current of the Renuvion® device is an order of magnitude lower. The current of the Renuvion® waveform flows through the conductive plasma beam to create additional beneficial Joule heating of the target tissue. However, since the current is so low, it is dispersed before it is able to penetrate deep into the tissue. This allows for soft tissue heating with minimal depth of thermal effect. This low current also prevents the tissue from being overtreated when subjected to multiple treatment passes. As the tissue is treated, it coagulates and desiccates resulting in an increase in tissue impedance. The lower current of the Renuvion® device is unable to push through higher impedance tissue. As the Renuvion® device passes in proximity to previously

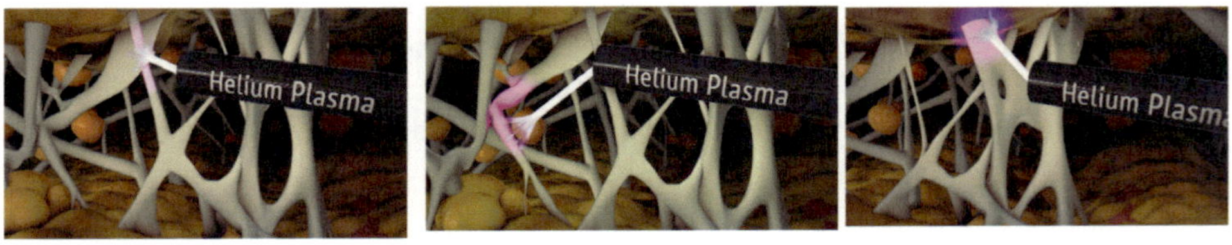

Figure 7.
The Renuvion® plasma beam quickly alternates between treating the different tissues surrounding the tip of the device. Instead of treating all tissue in the field, the approach is fractional. By targeting low impedance targets, tissue shrinks well without excessive heating.

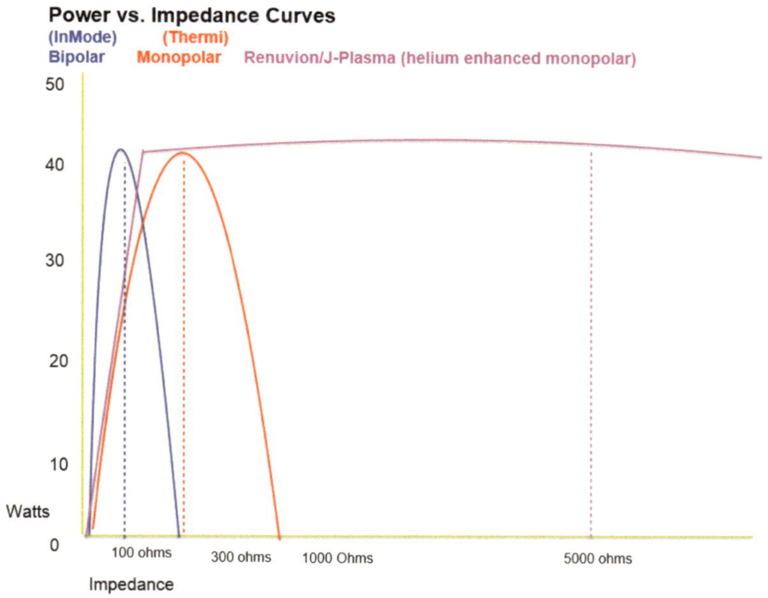

Figure 8.
Output power vs. impedance curves for subdermal energy devices.

treated tissue, the energy will follow the path of least resistance (lower impedance) and preferentially treat previously untreated tissue. This prevents overtreating of any one particular area with multiple passes and maximizes the treatment of untreated tissue. **Figure 8** shows a comparison of power versus impedance curves for bulk heating devices versus the plasma fractional RF device.

8.5 Renuvion®—helium

Although other inert gases can and have been used in plasma devices for medical applications, the Renuvion® device uses helium due to its unique properties which translate into certain clinical advantages. Helium has a simple molecular structure consisting of only two electrons. This simple structure allows helium to be ionized using very low input of energy. The ionization of helium is therefore very controlled and produces a precise and stable output of energy. Helium facilitates the use of the low-current, proprietary RF waveform from the Renuvion® generator.

In summary, the Renuvion® helium-based plasma device from Bovie Medical has technological features that result in a unique and effective method of action for subdermal coagulation and contraction of soft tissue. These features are as follows:

1. The Renuvion® device achieves soft tissue coagulation and contraction by rapidly heating the treatment site to temperatures greater than 85°C for between 0.040 and 0.080 s [15].

2. The tissue surrounding the treatment site remains at much cooler temperatures resulting in rapid cooling after the application of the energy through conductive heat transfer.

3. Focused delivery of energy on immediate heating of the FSN resulting in immediate soft tissue contraction without unnecessarily heating the full thickness of the dermis.

4. 360° tissue treatment without the need for the user to redirect the flow of energy due to electrical energy taking the path of least resistance.

5. Unencumbered delivery of power regardless of the tissue impedance due to the unique power output from the electrosurgical generator.

6. Low-current RF energy resulting in minimal depth of thermal effect and prevention of overtreating tissue when performing multiple passes.

9. Indications

Indications for treatment with plasma-driven RF include focal lipodystrophy with mild to moderate soft tissue laxity. Post-bariatric patients can be treated if the need for skin contraction is less than 33% and if pendulosity of the tissue is mild. If the patient's focus is skin quality without excision, or improvement in poor soft tissue tone, the addition of this energy can improve outcomes. Patients who have given birth and want to restore their physique can also be helped, but diastasis recti can only be slightly improved with subcutaneous RF stimulation of the lax fascia. Breast lifting can be achieved to a significant degree, but the technique works best in patients with grade I and II ptosis and size C cup or less. The addition of a suspension suture can improve the outcome, especially for the subareolar and lower pole contour. Other popular treatment regions include the lower face and neck, upper arms, axilla, bra roll, abdomen and pubis, flanks, and circumferential thighs and knees.

10. Contraindications

Patients who should not be treated include:

1. Women who are pregnant or breastfeeding

2. Those with unrealistic expectations

3. Patients with an open sore in the treatment region

4. Patients with compromised healing such as oxygen dependence, diabetes if poorly controlled, and autoimmune disease

5. Severe pendulosity or skin/soft tissue laxity in the treatment region

6. Patients with significant skin compromise such as striae, scars, scleroderma, or lupus

7. Patients with previous treatments in the region of focus, thick or depressed scars, or poorly vascularized tissue

11. Operative technique

Patients are marked in an upright position. Depressions are marked, and protuberances are highlighted. The patient is asked to look down and note what she or he sees as the most important set of goals as far as fat reduction and skin tightening. This perspective may be somewhat different from the evaluating surgeon's view.

Steps in treatment include evaluation and marking, sterile prep and drape, and administration of anesthesia, which always includes tumescent infusion and can also include oral sedation, IV sedation, or general anesthesia. Liposuction, if indicated, of the treatment region is then performed. Treatment with subcutaneous heating of the Renuvion device follows. "Strokes" are considered as an insertion and slow withdrawal of the device. Ideally, the speed of withdrawal should be about 1.5 cm/s. A "pass" is considered to be a series of strokes performed from a single access point at the same depth. Lab studies show that in the typical treatment region, a series of three multidepth passes is required in order to see significant soft tissue and skin contraction within 24 h. In areas with a small surface area or limited amount of localized fat, two passes may be sufficient. Of course, in regions where adipose thickness is 3 cm or more, up to five passes at multiple depths may be needed in order to achieve the optimal outcome. Unless the treatment region is very thick, more than five passes in one region may be overtreatment.

Clinical endpoints with the Renuvion device are different from those with bulk heating treatment. There will be little localized warmth or erythema, because it is not a bulk heating device. A visible contraction of the skin surface with the handpiece slightly angled up upon withdrawal is an indicator of good response. Because there is not an energy expended measurement on the current generator, a good indicator is activated time on the tissue. I usually treat a 10 × 15 cm segment of the tissue with 5 kJ, which correlates to 5 min of handpiece activation time per region.

Some controversy exists regarding "cross-hatching" or creating a perpendicular series of passes in the same treatment zone. Because the device seeks out low impedance tissue to briefly heat, the "woven" or "crisscross" method is not routinely needed. However, in large areas or in regions needing optimal soft tissue contraction, this approach is recommended.

Cross-hatching is contraindicated in areas such as the lower face, jowls, jawline, submentum, or decollete. Thin upper arm skin may also not need two perpendicular approaches.

Treatment depths generally include the deep suprafascial zone, the midlevel of the adipose layer which corresponds to Scarpa's fascia, and the immediate subdermal region. In patients with thin skin, striae, or a previous procedure in the treatment zone, a conservative two layer approach is recommended. In necks, a supraplatysmal and a subdermal approach are recommended.

Multiple treatment levels are recommended to reduce the amount of adipose gliding that is seen with age, a decrease in the stromal collagen binding of fat, and hormonal change [37].

Patients who note a disconnection of the soft tissue from the rectus fascia when leaning forward can gain some readherence with multilevel treatment. Suprafascial heating of the abdominal midline can decrease diastasis recti up to 1 cm. Further studies are needed to show the duration of this response.

Enhancement of tissue response can be achieved by reducing local impedance with infusion of tumescent fluid and by removing the insulating adipose tissue. Undertumescing will decrease tissue response. An infusion ratio of 1:1 is recommended for most regions. By optimizing treatment temperature, the stromal fibrous collagen bands will contract more intensely and more quickly. A variety of optimal temperatures are shown in the biomechanical literature, ranging from 60 to 80°C. At lower temperatures, tissue contraction is slower. Perfusion is the most influential factor, as well as the most difficult to measure and influence. Good perfusion can be enhanced by avoiding overtumescing as the closing venous pressure will be exceeded. Using warm fluid is helpful. Vasodilators are not indicated. Perfusion can be compromised by mechanical factors such as tissue location in a fibrous area (flanks and bra roll). A frequently overlooked consideration is treatment in secondary cases. The presence of scar tissue in a patient who has undergone a previous procedure should be noted. The use of another energy-based device prior to the use of the primary heating device adds risk, such as liposuction using PAL or Vaser.

It is important to consider the effect of adding pressurized gas when treating the secondary patient. Fibrosis, whether induced by previous minimally invasive procedures or by surgery, will change the direction of the gas, which will follow the path of least resistance. While not clinically dangerous, the creation of temporary subcutaneous crepitus can be disconcerting to the patient. Careful and thorough tunneling of the treatment region will allow for gas egress in these cases. The use of more than one access port is imperative. Tunnels should be created in such a way that they communicate with one another, and aspiration of gas at the end of the procedure will improve patient comfort.

12. Results

Significant improvement in the contour and pendulosity of skin and soft tissue has been seen with the combination of liposuction and helium plasma-driven radiofrequency energy.

Interestingly, clinical endpoints are different with this device compared with bulk heaters. Because the skin does not heat up in broad regions, neither erythema nor warmth at the treatment site is an indicator of a completed treatment. However, early improvement can be seen as early as the next day.

While the presence of some fat in the neck to be treated with bulk heating devices is desired, it is not necessary when using the Renuvion device. **Figure 9** shows a 49-year-old woman with no fat in her neck preoperatively. A nice correction of her skin laxity is seen at 2 months post-op.

Figure 10 shows a 37-year-old man with gynecomastia and abdominal lipodystrophy. The device is quite good for treating larger surface areas on men or women, as the rapid heating of soft tissue has been shown to decrease overall operative time. Good definition without contour irregularities is noted postoperatively.

The use of energy-based devices has been somewhat limited in the older patient. Because both skin quality and cohesiveness of the subcutaneous tissue can be compromised, these patients are usually offered excisional procedures. **Figure 11**

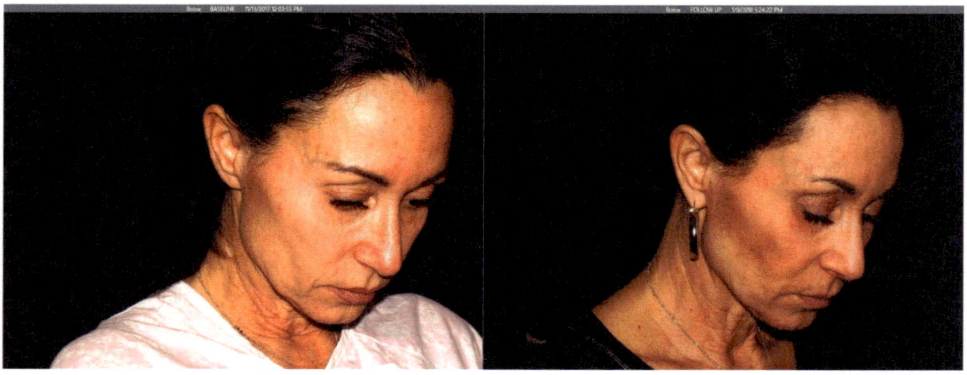

(a) (b)

Figure 9.
(a) A 49-year-old patient with neck laxity and (b) a patient 2 months following tumescent infusion and subcutaneous heating with Renuvion. No liposuction was performed.

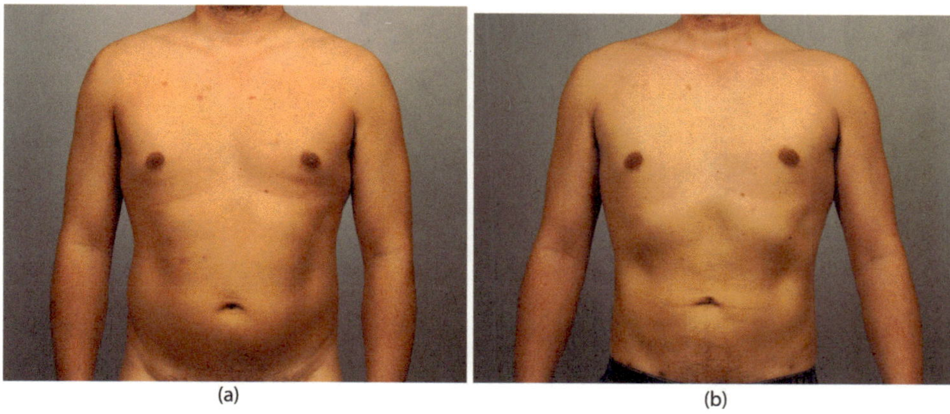

Figure 10.
(a) A 37-year-old man with lipodystrophy of the abdomen, flanks, and chest and (b) a patient 3 months post treatment with liposuction and Renuvion soft tissue heating.

shows a 65-year-old woman who underwent circumferential liposuction and Renuvion RF tightening. She has excellent reduction of the skin envelope with improvement of skin tone and texture.

Figure 12 shows a 37-year-old man who had multiple areas of lipodystrophy, despite an active job. He was treated with liposuction and helium-driven plasma RF tightening of the fibroseptal network in the chest, abdomen, and flank region. New technology shows the directional lift achieved in the lower abdomen that corrects the preoperative pendulosity. Skin compression diagram shows relative tightening of the skin in the treatment region (**Figure 13**).

13. Risk reduction in energy-assisted lipocontouring

Side effects can be seen when using any energy-based device. With radiofrequency, most of these are thermal. There is a difference between expected sequelae and adverse sequelae.

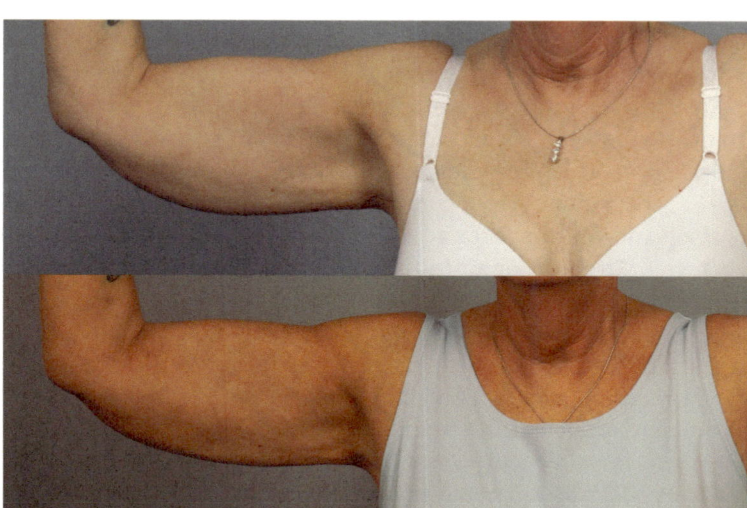

Figure 11.
A 65-year-old woman with pendulosity of the volar upper arm (above). Below, a patient 3 months after circumferential liposuction and treatment with Renuvion. Pendulosity measurement decreased by 40%.

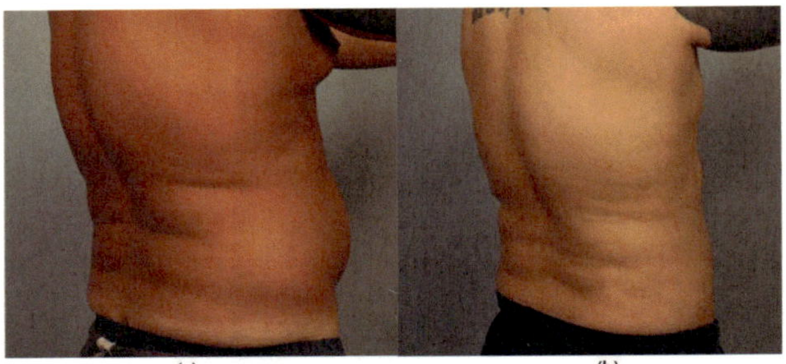

Figure 12.
This 38-year-old man had gynecomastia, abdominal lipodystrophy with pendulosity, and flank and waist fatty hyperplasia and tissue contraction at 6 weeks. (a) A patient before treatment and (b) a patient 6 weeks after liposuction plus Renuvion.

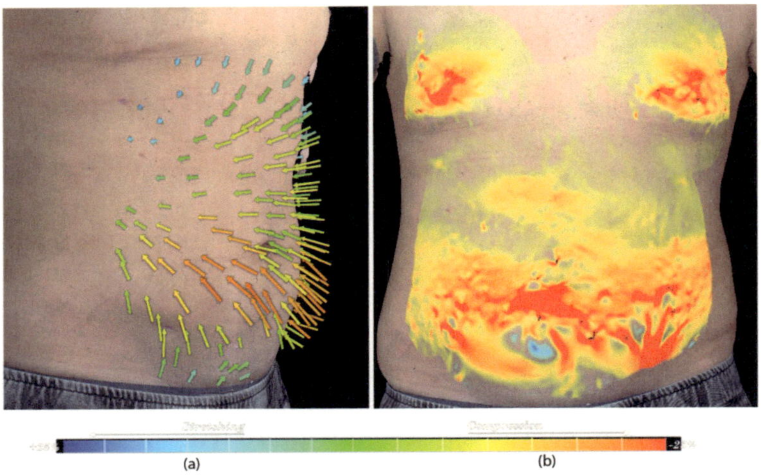

Figure 13.
(a) Postoperative analysis of directional lift following liposuction and Renuvion RF assisted tissue tightening. (b) Compressive tissue analysis of the same patient following treatment with abdominal liposuction and Renuvion tissue tightening.

Expected sequelae include erythema, swelling, and redness and small scar at the access port sites. Bruising may be prolonged, and a temporarily modest improvement due to post-op swelling is expected. Patients may note they cannot fit into their regular size of clothing for a few weeks. Less than hoped for improvement in the early weeks is expected. Tissue contraction really becomes noticeable about 3 months post-op and continues for a year or more. Pre-existing asymmetry will not be totally corrected. Crepitus or air in the tissue due to residual helium is common, even if gas is expressed or suctioned at case end.

Adverse sequelae can include persistent tissue pendulosity if present preoperatively. Creases or folds in the skin can occur if the patient is not careful about compression garment application. Small burns or blistering can occur but this is rare. If heat or ice is applied to the treatment region postoperatively, an area of full-thickness skin loss can occur. Unsatisfactory scarring at the access port sites may occur. Rarely, fibrosis can occur in overtreated regions. Undertreatment may result in residual lipodystrophy, a hooded umbilicus, or focal skin contour irregularities.

These irregularities can also occur if fat pad thickness is not checked for uniformity prior to closure. Overly aggressive liposuction, especially if superficial, can leave an unattractive skin surface.

Top 10 technical tips for achieving good outcomes:

1. Use DocMatter. The device company has set up a discussion forum, DocMatter. This website is easily accessible and promotes an open review of techniques and outcomes.

2. Initial assessment is critical. If the patient has a significant diastasis recti or needs more than 33% skin contraction, especially in a localized area, the treating physician should explain the limitations of a minimally invasive approach.

3. Treatment of multiple tissue layers is important. Dr. Sonja Sattler notes that the soft tissue regions have a gliding aspect in which the skin and superficial fat become disconnected with the deep fascia with aging. When performing abdominoplasty, I have noted that many patients have very little attachment of the deep fat to rectus fascia. Therefore, in order to reconnect the soft tissue to underlying fascia, it is optimal to treat several levels—suprafascial, midlevel, or Scarpa's fascia and the immediate subdermal fat—with the Renuvion device. Clinical laboratory studies show that 3–4 passes (several ray-type strokes in a given region) will give optimal soft tissue and skin shrinkage in the average treatment region.

4. In regions with less fat, such as the neck, decollete, some arms, knees, and lower faces, only two levels of treatment are needed. Less is more here.

5. Because the current iteration of Renuvion does not measure energy expended, it can be difficult to understand the clinical endpoint. Clinical lab studies have shown that 1 min of activated handpiece time on the tissue is equivalent to 1 kJ of energy. If a 10 × 15 cm region is demarcated, an average of 5 min time on the tissue is optimal. This is equivalent to about a hand-sized region.

6. In regions where the skin is thin, less energy is needed. In the neck and jawline, 3–5 kJ total is recommended. A region of risk is the central cervicomental angle. By marking this area, and avoiding repeated passes, the risk of a burn is diminished.

7. Compression is king. Patients are informed that the best outcomes are obtained when a team approach is adopted. The surgeon can only influence the outcome during the surgical procedure and in the office during postoperative visits. It is the patient's responsibility to perform proper aftercare. By utilizing serially smaller compression garments and kinesiology tape where indicated, the desired smooth contour can be optimized.

8. Dr. Adam Rubenstein notes that patient selection is the most important aspect of treatment. Choosing a patient with a mild to moderate amount of subcutaneous fat and associated skin laxity is key. Managing expectations should be done at the outset in order to avoid postoperative disappointment. By reminding the patient that minimally invasive procedures cannot achieve the degree of change seen with skin excision, patient understanding of expected outcomes is optimized.

9. Dr. Ed Zimmerman recommends venting the access port not in use with a 1 cc syringe and plunger removed. This saves time as little gas is retained.

10. Dr. Gerhard Sattler likes to use a bit more tumescent fluid in a secondary treatment, as well as the PAL handpiece. This approach optimizes tunneling though fibrous tissue and allows for more thorough liposuction, tissue protection from overtreatment, and creation of regions of low impedance recipient tissue.

14. Conclusion

The use of helium-driven plasma energy is a new and promising resource for achieving non-excisional soft tissue and skin tightening. The use of the device for skin tightening is off label. This versatile treatment can be used in multiple regions, and its safety profile is strong. Because the subcutaneous fibroseptal network is the treatment target, there is no real focus on heating overlying skin. Clinical FLIR measurements show that in an average treatment region, skin temperatures get to about 38° when treated with Renuvion, as opposed to 45° and higher with bulk heating devices. Because the device rapidly heats a small segment of subcutaneous collagen to 85°C, strong immediate contraction is generated within 0.044 s. A rapid post-liposuction tissue treatment is followed by very visible improvement at the 24 h post-op mark. Results can continue to improve over a year, as infiltration of new collagen within the adipose stroma occurs. Restoration of the adipose framework can recreate a firm rather than flabby feel of the soft tissue, along with a defined shape.

Author details

Diane Irvine Duncan
Private Practice, Fort Collins, Colorado

*Address all correspondence to: momsurg@aol.com

References

[1] Bellini E, Grieco MP, Raposio E. A journey through liposuction and liposculture: Review. Annals of Medicine and Surgery. 2017;**24**:53-60. DOI: 10.1016/j.amsu.2017.10.024

[2] Illouz Y. Body contouring by lipolysis: A 5 year experience with over 3000 cases. Plastic and Reconstructive Surgery. 1983;**72**:511

[3] Kesselring LK, Meyer R. A suction curette for removal of excessive local deposits of subcutaneous fat. Plastic and Reconstructive Surgery. 1978;**62**:305

[4] Fischer A, Fischer G. First surgical treatment for molding body's cellulite with three 5 mm incisions. Bulletin of the International Academy of Cosmetic Surgery. 1976;**3**:35

[5] Illouz YG. History and current concepts of lipoplasty. Clinics in Plastic Surgery. 1996;**23**:721-730

[6] Klein JA. Tumescent technique for local anesthesia. The Western Journal of Medicine. 1996;**164**(6):517

[7] Klein JA, Jeske DR. Estimated maximal safe dosages of tumescent lidocaine. Anesthesia and Analgesia. 2016;**122**(5):1350-1359

[8] Sattler G, Eichner S. Complications of liposuction. Der Hautarzt. 2013; **64**(3):171-179. DOI: 10.1007/s00105-012-2487-8

[9] Iverson RE, Lynch DJ. American Society of Plastic Surgeons Committee on Patient Safety. Practice advisory on liposuction. Plastic and Reconstructive Surgery. 2004;**113**(5):1478-1490, discussion 1491-5

[10] Sumrall AJ. A review of liposuction as a cosmetic surgical procedure. Journal of the National Medical Association. 1987;**79**:1275-1279

[11] Maxwell GP, Gingrass MK. Ultrasound-assisted lipoplasty: A clinical study of 250 consecutive patients. Plastic and Reconstructive Surgery. 1998;**101**:189-202, discussion 203

[12] DiBernardo BE, Reyes J. Evaluation of skin tightening after laser-assisted liposuction. Aesthetic Surgery Journal. 2009;**29**:400-407

[13] Fodor PB. Power-assisted lipoplasty versus traditional suction-assisted lipoplasty: Comparative evaluation and analysis of output. Aesthetic Plastic Surgery. 2005;**29**(2):127

[14] Man D, Meyer H. Water jet-assisted lipoplasty. Aesthetic Surgery Journal. 2007;**27**:342-346

[15] Kiełczewska M, Szymczyk J, Leszczyńsk R, Błaszczyk. The effect of high-frequency current and ultrasonic wave on selected indicators of body weight. Polski Merkuriusz Lekarski. 2015;**38**(225):150-154

[16] Blugerman G, Schavelzon D, Paul MD. A safety and feasibility study of a novel radiofrequency-assisted liposuction technique. Plastic and Reconstructive Surgery. 2010;**125**: 998-1006

[17] Paul M, Mulholland RS. A new approach for adipose tissue treatment and body contouring using radiofrequency-assisted liposuction. Aesthetic Plastic Surgery. 2009;**33**: 687-694

[18] Rubin JP, Khachi G. Mastopexy after massive weight loss: Dermal suspension and selective auto-augmentation. Clinics in Plastic Surgery. 2008;**35**(1):123-129. Review

[19] Cotofana S, Fratila AA, Schenck TL, Redka-Swoboda W, Zilinsky I, Pavicic T.

The anatomy of the aging face: A review. Facial Plastic Surgery. 2016;**32**(3): 253-260. DOI: 10.1055/s-0036-1582234. Epub 2016 Jun 1

[20] Watanabe M, Buch K, Fujita A, Christiansen CL, Jara H, Sakai O. MR relaxometry for the facial ageing assessment: The preliminary study of the age dependency in the MR relaxometry parameters within the facial soft tissue. Dento Maxillo Facial Radiology. 2015;**44**(7):20150047. DOI: 10.1259/dmfr.20150047

[21] Szczerkowska-Dobosz A, Olszewska B, Lemańska M, Purzycka-Bohdan D, Nowicki R. Acquired facial lipoatrophy: Pathogenesis and therapeutic options. Postepy Dermatologii i Alergologii. 2015;**32**(2):127-133

[22] Duncan DI. Aging Adipose Tissue in Skin Types I-VI: Scanning Electron Micrograph Analysis. Paris, France: IMCAS Paris; 2015

[23] Duncan Duncan DI. Nonexcisional tissue tightening: Creating skin surface area reduction during abdominal liposuction by adding radiofrequency heating. Aesthetic Surgery Journal. 2013;**33**(8):1154-1166

[24] Zocchi M. Ultrasonic liposculpturing. Aesthetic Plastic Surgery. 1992;**16**:287-298

[25] Key DJ. A preliminary study of a transdermal radiofrequency device for body slimming. Journal of Drugs in Dermatology. 2015;**14**(11):1272-1278

[26] Duncan DI. Improving outcomes in upper arm liposuction: Adding radiofrequency-assisted liposuction to induce skin contraction. Aesthetic Surgery Journal. 2012;**32**(1):84-95

[27] Landen N, Li D, Stahle M. Transition from inflammation to proliferation: A critical step during wound healing. Cellular and Molecular Life Sciences. 2016;**73**(20):3861-3885

[28] Toledo LS. Syringe liposculpture. Clinics in Plastic Surgery. 1996;**23**: 683-693

[29] Hughes CE 3rd. Reduction of lipoplasty risks and mortality: An ASAPS survey. Aesthetic Surgery Journal. 2001;**21**:120-127

[30] Duncan DI, Kreindel M. Basic radiofrequency: Physics and safety and application to aesthetic medicine. In: Lapidoth M, Halachmi S, editors. Radiofrequency in Cosmetic Dermatology, Aesthet Dermatol. Vol. 2. Basel: Karger; 2015. pp. 1-22

[31] Huang G, Li F, Zhao X, Ma Y, Li Y, Lin M, et al. Genin functional and biomimetic materials for engineering of the three-dimensional cell microenvironment. Chemical Reviews. 2017;**117**(20):12764-12850. DOI: 10.1021/acs.chemrev.7b00094

[32] Arunachalam SP, Rossman PJ, Arani A, Lake DS, Glaser KJ, Trzasko JD, et al. Quantitative 3D magnetic resonance elastography: Comparison with dynamic mechanical analysis. Magnetic Resonance in Medicine. 2017;**77**(3): 1184-1192. DOI: 10.1002/mrm.26207. Epub 2016 Mar 26

[33] Duck FA. Physical Properties of Tissue. London: Academic Press Limited; 1990

[34] Thomsen S. Pathologic analysis of photothermal and photomechanical effects of laser-tissue interactions. Photochemistry and Photobiology. 1991; **53**:825-835

[35] Massarweh NN, Cosgriff N, Slakey DP. Electrosurgery: History, principles, and current and future uses. Journal of the American College of Surgeons. 2006;**202**(3):520-530

[36] Hurwitz D, Smith D. Treatment of overweight patients by radiofrequency-assisted liposuction (RFAL) for aesthetic reshaping and skin tightening. Aesthetic Plastic Surgery. 2012;**36**(1): 62-71

[37] Sattler G, Sommer B, Bergfeld D, Sattler S. Tumescent liposuction in Germany: History and new trends and techniques. Dermatologic Surgery. 1999; **25**(3):221-223

Chapter 4

BodyTite®: The Science and Art of Radiofrequency Assisted Lipocoagulation (RFAL) in Body Contouring Surgery

Robert Stephen Mulholland

Abstract

BodyTite® is a bipolar, radiofrequency assisted lipocoagulation (RFAL) system and concept that helps the liposuction surgeon better control soft tissue contraction and the contours of the face, neck and body when performing aspiration lipoplasty, or skin tightening alone. There are several different BodyTite® hand pieces that are designed for different clinical procedures and body contouring applications. This chapter outlines the basic science of RFAL, the scientific evidence for contraction and efficacy, as well as, the authors 10-year experience using BodyTite® and RFAL hand pieces to deliver the best possible soft tissue contraction and body contouring.

Keywords: radiofrequency-assisted liposuction/lipocoagulation, RFAL, liposuction, body sculpting, body contouring, BodyTite®, FaceTite®, AccuTite and CelluTite

1. Introduction

Liposuction is the most common cosmetic plastic surgery procedure in the world. The advent of tumescent microcannula suction-assisted lipoplasty (SAL) technique, Power-assisted lipoplasty (PAL), ultrasound-assisted lipoplasty (UAL or Vaser), water-assisted lipoplasty (WAL), laser-assisted lipoplasty (LAL, or SmartLipo) have all been energy assisted innovations to the liposuction technique that have contributed to making liposuction less traumatic, faster, optimize the extraction technique with stem cell preservation (UAL) or offer moderate dermal contraction (LAL) [1–6]. Despite these advances in the basic liposuction technique, one of the major challenges facing liposuction surgeons is optimizing and ensuring soft tissue contraction and body contouring outcomes after removal of adipose tissue [7–11]. Worsening of skin laxity and suboptimal soft tissue contraction following adipose aspiration is common [1].

The Introduction of BodyTite® Radiofrequency Assisted Liposuction 10 years ago and the evolution of the various RFAL applicators and technology since that time has led to an era of optimal control of soft tissue contraction and more consistency in quality body contouring results [12–14]. This chapter outlines the peer reviewed articles and basic science of BodyTite® and reviews the authors use of RFAL in over 1000 cases in his body contouring and facial rejuvenation practice.

IntechOpen

2. Basic science of BodyTite® and RFAL

The BodyTite® device is comprised of a workstation, or platform, which houses the RF Generator, software and circuit boards of the system. Into this workstation attach the various clinic hand pieces (**Figure 1**). The hand pieces come in different sizes and configurations and are designed for specific clinical procedures and anatomical locations.

Each BodyTite® hand piece is in a bipolar configuration, where the internal electrode is a silicon coated cannula that is RF emitting in its distal uncoated region and has a sophisticated bullet shaped tip to aid is soft tissue dissection and movement, while minimizing the risk of end dermal hits and thermal injury.

The external electrode, which is attached to the same hand piece, slides along the surface of the skin in tandem with the internal electrode (**Figure 2**).

The internal electrode emits positively charged RF current, which flows back and forth from the positively charged internal electrode to the negatively charged external electrode. The RF is strongly ablative and coagulative within 1–2 cm of the internal electrode and dissipates at is flows and diffuses up to the external electrode. Soft tissue within 1–2 cm of the internal electrode will undergo a necrotic, ablative tissue thermal effect, while the dermis will experience a sub-necrotic, non- ablative dermal, thermal stimulation.

The Radiofrequency energy within 1–2 cm of the internal electrode provides a coagulative, ablative issue on local tissue, adipose, vascular and the fibroseptal network (FSN). As RF flows up, ever more diffusely, to the external electrode moving in parallel and in tandem with the internal electrode, RF will be more diffuse and is flowing to a much broader, bigger surface area electrode and the thermal effect on the dermal structures will be non-ablative heating (**Figure 3**).

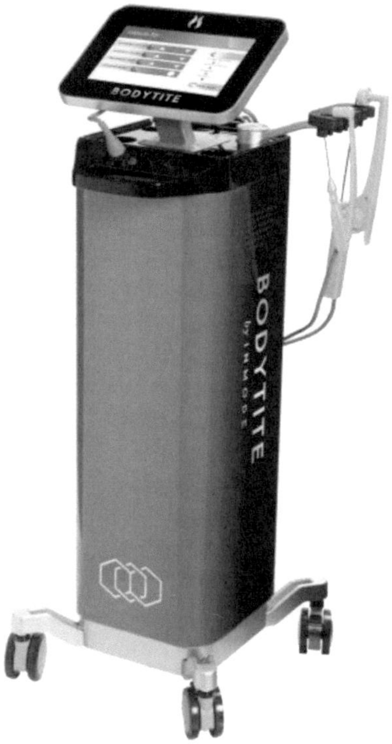

Figure 1.
The BodyTite® RFAL workstation. The various hand pieces in the BodyTite® RFAL family plug into the workstation.

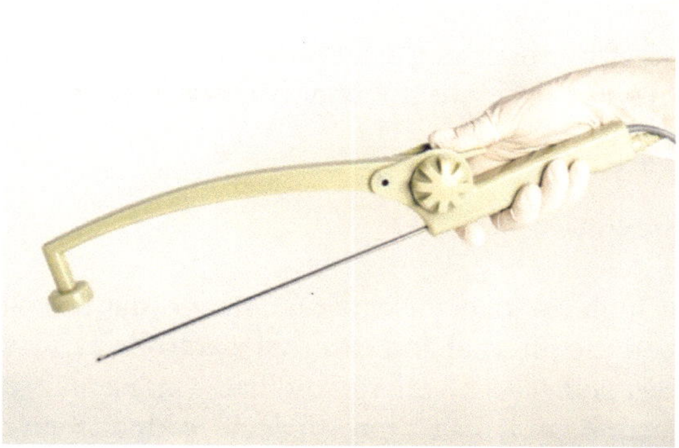

Figure 2.
The BodyTite® bipolar RFAL hand piece.

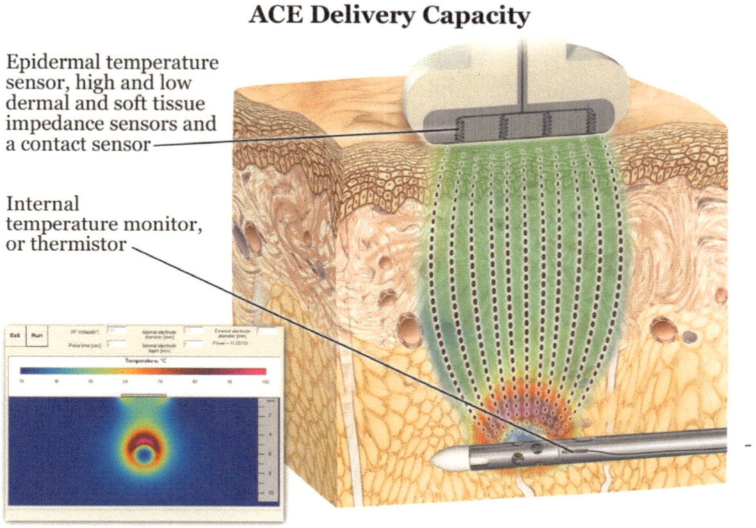

Figure 3.
The RF energy flows from the internal electrode, where it is ablative in nature, to the external electrode, where the RF has a gentle non-ablative thermal effect on the dermis.

The Soft tissue tightening concept of BodyTite® is to provide and 3-dimensional contraction of the soft tissue through internal RF stimulation and contraction of the Fibroseptal network, together with dermal enhancement through non-ablative thermal stimulation and neo-collagenases [15].

2.1 Safety features of the BodyTite® hand pieces

The Following features have been built into the hardware and software of the BodyTite® to optimize soft tissue contraction and minimize the risk of a thermal injury.

2.1.1 The silastic coating and cap

The proximal internal electrode is silicone coated along its length to minimize the risk of a thermal injury to the access port and soft tissue that is not in direct proximity to the tip. There is a small, distal section of the internal electrode that is not silicon coated and this portion emits the positive charged radiofrequency energy. The distal aspect of the internal electrode has a silastic, bullet shaped cap, which facilitates dissection through the adipose tissue and minimizes the risk of an end dermal hit, or thermal injury to the underside of the dermis or deeper, delicate soft tissue structures.

2.1.2 Thermal containment

The RF energy is high frequency electrical current that travels in a wave form and oscillates between the internal and external electrode at a frequency of 1 million cycles per second. The RF energy oscillates molecular structures in its path 1 million time per second, generating intermolecular kinetic energy and heat. The heat can be necrotic and ablative in nature (near the tip) or sub necrotic, non-ablative tissue heating (the external electrode). The RF flows from the small, internal electrode with a smaller, more focused tip and high power density to the larger, lower power density external electrode providing "thermal containment", or heating energy between the two electrodes, with very little heating below the internal electrode, which is a safety feature when performing RFAL around delicate structures like the face and neck where there is a the Facial nerve that is under the investing fascia of the facial muscles and is sensitive to thermal stimulation if there were significant heat flowing below the internal electrode.

2.1.3 Automate feedback control loops

There are a number of high-tech sensors built into the BodyTite® hand pieces that communicate with the software algorithm on the workstation (**Figure 4**).

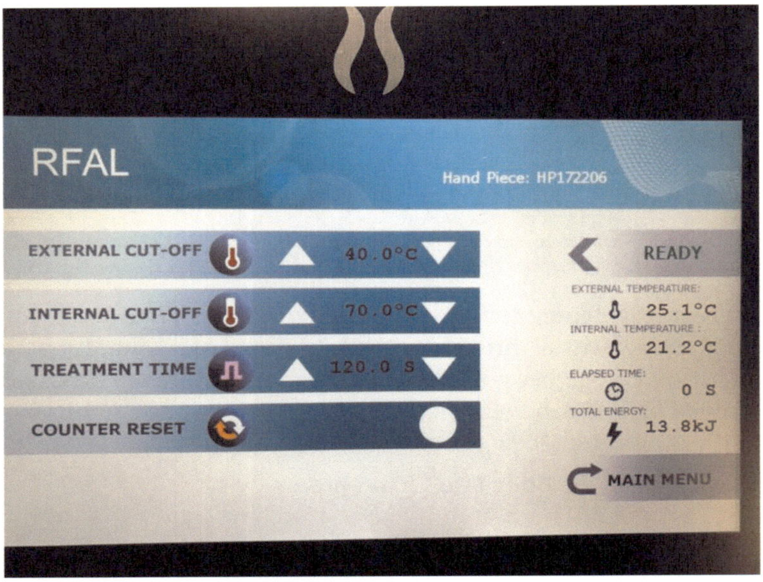

Figure 4.
The GUI screen o the BodyTite® RFAL workstation. On the left hand side, he external (skin) electrode and internal electrode (adipose) cut off temperatures are set by the physician. Increments of 120 s of RF energy are dispended and when the 120 s are up, double clicking on the foot pedal gives another 120 s. On the right-hand side are the real time temperatures of the external skin and internal fat temperatures as measured by the external electrode and internal electrode thermistors. As the user gets within 2°C of the cut off temperature, the audible beep that is emitted when RF energy is on, increases in tempo and when the cut off temperature is reached, either internal or external, the and audible will sound that is characteristic for the external and one for the internal cut-off and the RF energy delivered is terminated to the hand piece and tissue heating stops. When the external and internal temperature is 0.1°C below the cut-off RF energy flow begins again. The automated feedback loop allows heating of the adipose and skin to occur together or independently and not exceed the pre-set amounts.

Contact *Sensors:* within the external electrode there is a contact sensor and if there is loss of contact, the RF flow is cut-off, minimizing the risk of arch burns or excessive flow from the internal electrode. *External and Internal Thermistors:* there are thermistors in the external electrode and near the tip of the internal electrode (US models only) that continuously measure the local temperature every millisecond. The Thermistors permit the physician to enter the desired cut off temperature of the skin and internal cut off temperature of the adipose tissue and the software algorithm within the workstation will cut off the RF energy when the desired external or internal cut-off temperature is achieved. *Temperature Display and Audible Alerts*: the device interface displays the internal and external temperatures at all times and has an audible alert when the skin, or internal temperature is within 2°C of the cut-off and, then another distinct audible for the both the skin and internal temperature when the desired cut-off temperature has been reached. When the cut off temperature has been achieved the RF will be turn off and on again around that temperature, allowing the physician to sustain the desired thermal endpoint for a prolonged period of time, if desired.

The treatment time and amount of energy delivered in seconds and KJ is measured.

Impedance Cut offs: impedance is the resistance to RF flow through tissue. As the tissue temperature increases, impedance will decrease and if the impedance drop is too great, then the RF energy will be cut off. Conversely, if the resistance to flow is too great (usual cause is divergent electrodes, where the internal is going one way and the external another), or there is solid tissue between the electrodes, or very fibrous tissue between the two electrodes, the impedance will rise and the RF energy is cut off.

Temperature Surge Protection (TSP): the BodyTite® applicator and workstation will continuously measure the *"rate of rise of temperature"* and will deliver full RF power if the tissue is being heated at less than, or equal to 20°C/cm^3/s, but will decrease the RF energy if the rate of rise of temperature is between 20 and 35°C/cm^3/s until the rate of rise of temperature is again 20C/cm^3/s and will turn off the RF energy completely (necessitating stepping on the foot pedal again to start) if the rate of rise exceeds 35°C/cm^3/s, a process is called TSP, or Temperature Surge Protection, or TSP. This rate of rise of temperature algorithm is empirical and based upon the observations that excellent FSN shortening and soft tissue contraction can be achieved less than 20°, which the risk of thermal injury increases as more tissue is heated/cm^3/s. The physician does not select an energy setting or desired power when selecting treatment parameters, as the device will automatically give enough RF power to maintain a heating profile of 20°C/cm^3/s. The US version of the BodyTite® has TSP, while the International version does not and uses high and low internal impedance cut offs rather than TSP. The international version allows the physician to enter the desired power (up to 70 W for the larger BodyTite® hand pieces and 25 W for the smaller FaceTite® applicators and aspirates while it coagulates. as the internal electrode is a hollow cannula and the hand piece can hook up to wall suction. The US version is non-aspirating and all suction is performed after or before the RFAL a non-thermal SAL or PAL cannula.

2.2 Evidence for RFAL thermal contraction

There are a number of well-designed studies that have confirmed significant soft tissue contraction following BodyTite® and RFAL. Kreindel and Mulholland were able to show the vertical, horizontal and oblique fibers of FSN (**Figure 5**) as the major vehicle for significant three-dimensional soft tissue contraction at the time of surgery [15]. Further, this paper showed that 69° was the optimal temperature for thermal contraction and shortening of the FSN network. Duncan and others [16],

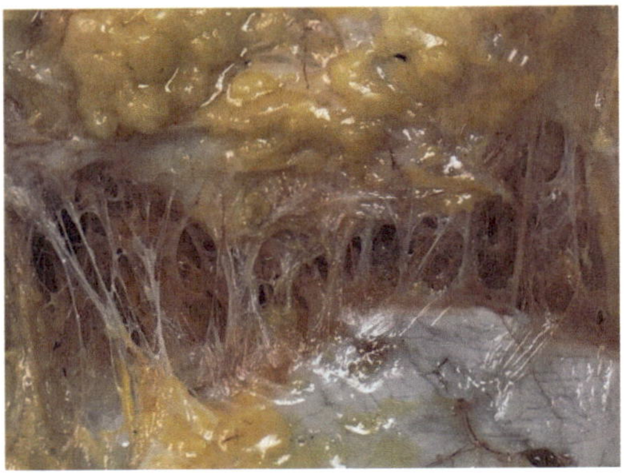

Figure 5.
The FSN are shown above connecting the anterior rectus sheet below to the overlying abdominal adipose tissue. The vertical, horizontal and oblique Fibroseptal bands will shorten and contract when the RFAL thermal temperature and stimulation reaches 69°C pulling the overlying soft tissue envelope in tighter association with the underlying muscle and delivering soft tissue contraction.

were able to confirm upwards of 25% soft tissue area contraction after BodyTite® and RFAL at 6 months, which increased to 34% at 12 months. There have been numerous clinical papers outlining the soft tissue contraction advantages of the RFAL applicators in the face, neck, arms, inner thighs and body [17–22].

3. Clinical approach and basic parameters

The basic RFAL approach of the author has been to deploy BodyTite® applicators just before aspiration to ensure optimal soft tissue contraction, liquefy the adipose tissue for more gentle aspiration forces and coagulate the small venules and arterioles to lessen post aspiration extravasation and ecchymosis. Some physicians choose to aspirate first and perform the RFAL after debulking and they have reported good results with this technique, but theoretically aspirating first may compromise and traumatize some of the FSN, perhaps limiting the amount of contraction that could occur and would injure the small vessels before thermal coagulation increasing the risk of bruising.

The BodyTite® applicators come with a dial on the hand piece that can control the distance between the internal and external electrodes, facilitating delivering thermal coagulation and different depths and levels. In general, Level 6, 5, 4, 3, 2 and 1 correspond to 6, 5, 4, 3, 2 and 1 cm inter-electrode distance and, remember, the effective coagulation is within 1–2 cm of the tip of the internal electrode (**Figure 6**).

3.1 The basic principles of RFAL treatment are

1. Shorten the vertical, oblique and horizontal FSN for optimal contraction.

2. **The FSN contracts** optimally at 69°C.

3. **The area of thermal coagulation** radiates within 1–2 cm of the uncoated tip of the internal electrode/cannula.

4. **Multiple, vertical sequential** levels of the adipose tissue will be needed to be treated to ensure optimal recruitment and coagulation of the FSN.

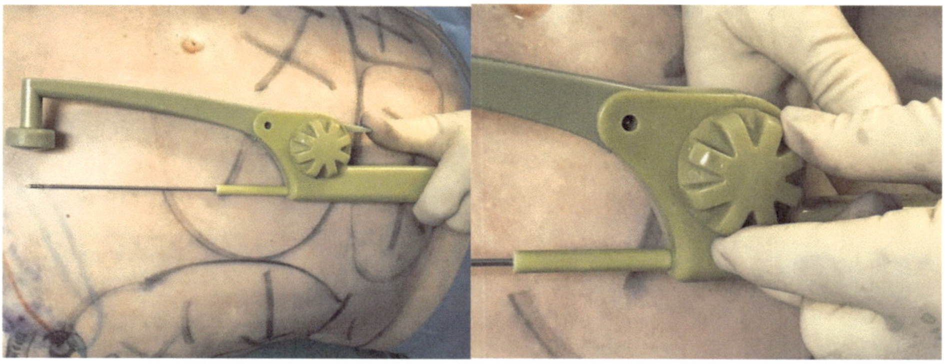

Figure 6.
The various BodyTite® applicators are bipolar RF electrodes, with the internal, positively charged electrode being inserted into the adipose tissue and the external, negatively charged electrode sliding along the surface of the skin in tandem with the internal. RF flows from the internal, uncoated electrode with the RF energy is ablative close to the electrode, up through the adipose to the dermis, skin and large diameter electrode where the RF is then more diffuse and non-ablative in nature. The physician can control the distance between the electrodes by setting the inter-electrode distance on the proximal end of the hand piece. Each setting, 1–6 on the dial corresponds approximately to the number of centimeters between the electrodes.

5. **The FSN thermal stimulation** is planned every 2 cm, so for thinner lipodystrophic zones, only two levels of sequential thermal coagulation may be required, while for larger adipose zones, three or more levels are needed.

6. **Pinch test:** prior to the Tumescent infiltration, pinch the thickness of the zone of fat you are treating. Divide this distance in half to determine the thickness of the adipose tissue. Calculate the number of 2 cm increments will fit into the final thickness of the flap and that will determine how many vertical levels will be treated. For example, a zone of fat to be treated measures 12 cm when pinched, means that the flap is 6 cm thick. Starting from the bottom, 2 cm intervals factors 3 time into 6 cm. So, the first lipocoagulation pass will be a level 6, followed by levels 4 and then a pass at level 2 (the effective coagulation zone is 2 cm). The author does not find the need to treat any closer to the skin than level 2. If the pinch test was 10 cm = a 5 cm flap = level 5 and level 3 would be deployed.

7. **Tumescent infiltration:** super wet is preferred over Wet, or tense tumescent and remember, RF travels most efficiently in a salinized environment. The author uses "double strength" Klein solution to salinate the adipose tissue, as the majority of BodyTite® RFAL is performed under local anesthesia and the thermal stimulation is more uncomfortable than SAL, UAL or PAL.

8. **Stamping and vertical sequential thermal treatment:** the author starts at the deepest calculated depth and advances from the port the most distal aspect of the zone. The hand piece is withdrawn the width of the external electrode and the thermal energy is applied until for 1–2 s or an audible pop (International Physician system) or until the audible internal cut off of 69° sounds. The foot is taken off the pedal and the hand piece is then withdrawn the distance of the external hand piece width and the process repeated. This is called the stamping technique (stationary until the endpoint is released) (**Figure** 7).

Other physicians will withdraw very, very slowly, allowing the temperate to rise to therapeutic cut off while withdrawing. GOAL of this step is to ensure as much of

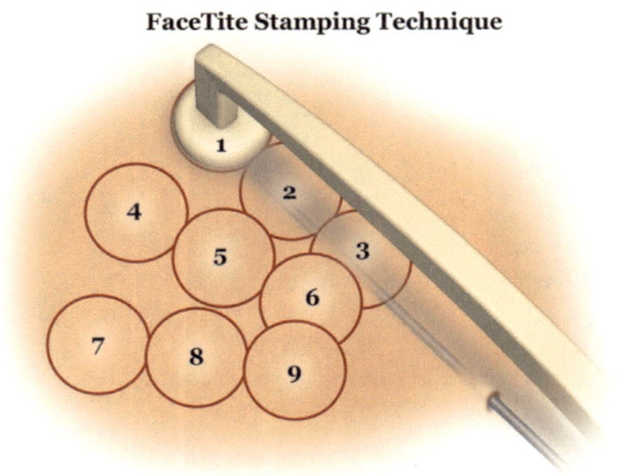

Figure 7.
The stamping technique. Stay in each spot until the internal thermal cut-off of 69–70 is reached, then move to the next spot.

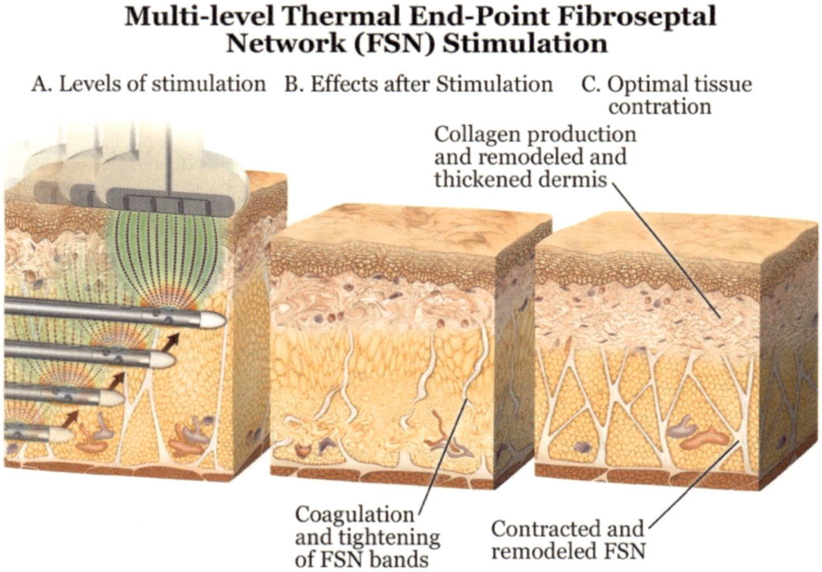

Figure 8.
Vertical sequential thermal stimulation to 69–70° cut-off is achieved, which is the temperature that optimizes the FSN contraction and remodeling, resulting in the 35% or greater skin and soft tissue contraction.

the FSN experiences 69°C for optimal contraction. This process is performed at each vertical levels determined by the "skin pinch" and 2 cm formula. Multiple, sequential vertical FSN thermal stimulation and contraction is then achieved, optimizing the 3D soft tissue skin and adipose contraction and body contouring results (**Figure 8**).

9. **Avoiding a peri-port burn: when you get close to the port, ensure you do** not end up at the same spot each time to avoid a peri-port burn. Try to zigzag through the adipose tissue as you advance and withdraw always to a different spot around the port (**Figure 9**).

Once I have stamped retrograde on the way back, or using a slow moving technique, I will keep my foot on the pedal and perform several back and forth

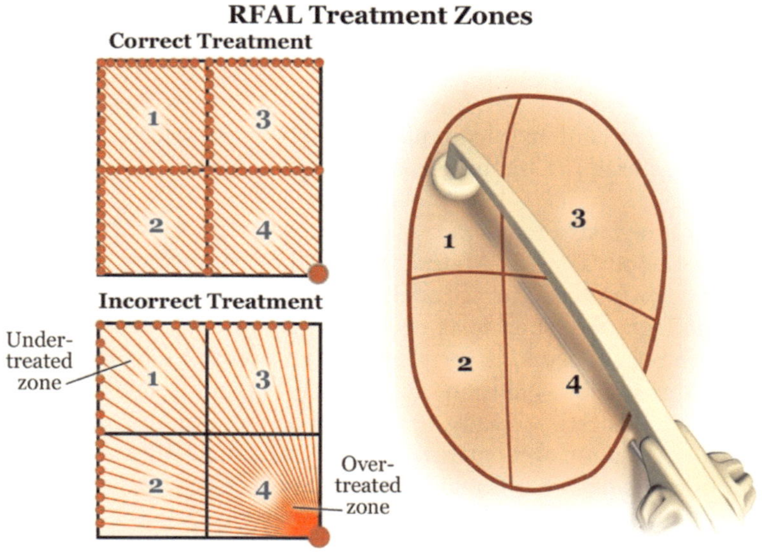

Figure 9.
Zig zag the applicator through the adipose tissue to avoid coming the same peri-port location each time, which will help avoid a peri-port thermal injury.

passes, slow moving technique, at that depth to ensure optimal thermal coverage of the FSN, as well as more complete lipocoagulation and liquification (easier aspiration, perhaps less trauma to the FSN, edema and pain) and coagulation of small venules and arterioles prior to aspiration (less ecchymosis). Again, it is important to zigzag your back stroke to avoid a peri-port burn (**Figure 9**).

10. When you have covered the 8 × 15 cm zone at one depth, stamping and slow moving, withdraw the internal electrode/cannula from the port and set the dial, 2 cm more superficial and repeat the stamping or slow withdrawing technique at the next, more superficial level. In the BodyTite® devices in the USA, the internal temperature before you move up to the next most superficial level must be 69 or 70° to get optimal FSN contraction (internal cut offs will not go higher the 70°). International BodyTite® users will find the external temperature will rise 4–5°C at each successive, more superficial level and there is no internal thermal cut-off control.

11. The skin temperature will continue to rise at each successive more superficial level until you approach the end point of 38–40°C. Both International and USA BodyTite® users would set their external skin cut off temperatures to 38–40°. *REMEMBER:* it is the FSN shortening that leads to the optimal soft tissue contraction, rather than non-ablative dermal heating. However, 38–40° epidermal, external cut off will result in more dermal collagen, elastin and ground substances, which will contribute to perhap. 15% over the overall tightening result, while FSN tightening accounts for 85% of the contraction we see with RFAL.

12. **Final aspiration and contouring:** when all levels have been treated and the adipose tissue has been heated to 69–70° and the skin to 38–40°, final aspiration is performed. International BodyTite® users have an aspirating internal electrode/cannula and this allows the physician to heat, coagulate and aspirate synchronously, so when they have completed the vertical sequential thermal coagulation, approximately 30% of the planned aspiration has

already been performed. It is more efficient to switch to dedicated aspirating cannulas or PAL systems when the thermal coagulation is done, than continue to aspirate with the RFAL cannula. United States BodyTite® users, have a non-aspirating cannula (FDA requirement) and suction begins once the vertical sequential thermal stimulation has been completed, again using dedicated aspiration cannula's or PAL systems.

13. **RFAL first or last?** From a purest perspective, there are advantages to performing BodyTite® RFAL first, followed by completion aspiration. However, some physician, particularly with larger BMI patients or large zones, perform the aspiration first, followed by BodyTite® thermal coagulation of the reduced, near final contour second (less tissue to heat) and perhaps refinement aspiration last. Although this approach is much faster, some of the theoretical disadvantages are: (i) more trauma to the FSN before thermal coagulation and potentially less contraction. (ii) traumatic aspiration disruption of small vessels may result in more ecchymosis, edema pain, hemosiderosis and hyperpigmentation.

3.2 Patient selection

Like any liposuction or Body Shaping procedure, RFAL patients need have realistic expectations, no uncontrolled medical conditions and appropriate skin tone and focal or multifocal lipodystrophy concerns. The BodyTite® family of applicators allow physicians to selection the right-hand piece for the job. International Physicians have a slightly different array of hand pieces and thermal controls than American physicians (FDA requirements) but both parameters are outlined below. In general, BodyTite® RFAL treatment can deliver up 35% area contraction over 12 months and, as such, does allow the physician to extend the indications for liposuction to patients with more skin laxity than they might have in the past. Those older patients, or those with larger BMI's, weight loss and weight gain, multiple parity may be BodyTite® candidates. The optimal RFAL soft tissue contraction means that physicians may be able to offer more minimal excisions: mini tummy tucks, axillary arm-lift, anterior inner thigh lifts and mini facelift in combination with BodyTite® RFAL treatment.

3.3 Port selection

Once you have selected a good BodyTite® candidate, then the appropriate port is selected to access the targeted lipocoagulation areas. Both RFAL BodyTite® and final aspiration contouring will be performed through the same port. Generally, this author prefers a single, well concealed port. The authors most favored zonal access ports are outlined in **Figure 10**.

3.4 RFAL thermal approach

Vertical sequential multi-level thermal coagulation, both stamping and/or slow moving to the deep (USA) and skin (International and USA) end points. Aspiration generally follows the heating (**Figure 8**).

3.5 Parameters

USA BodyTite® physicians: cut off of 69–70°C internal and 38–40°C external and 120 second treatment cycles. In the USA, the energy in watts is not entered as the

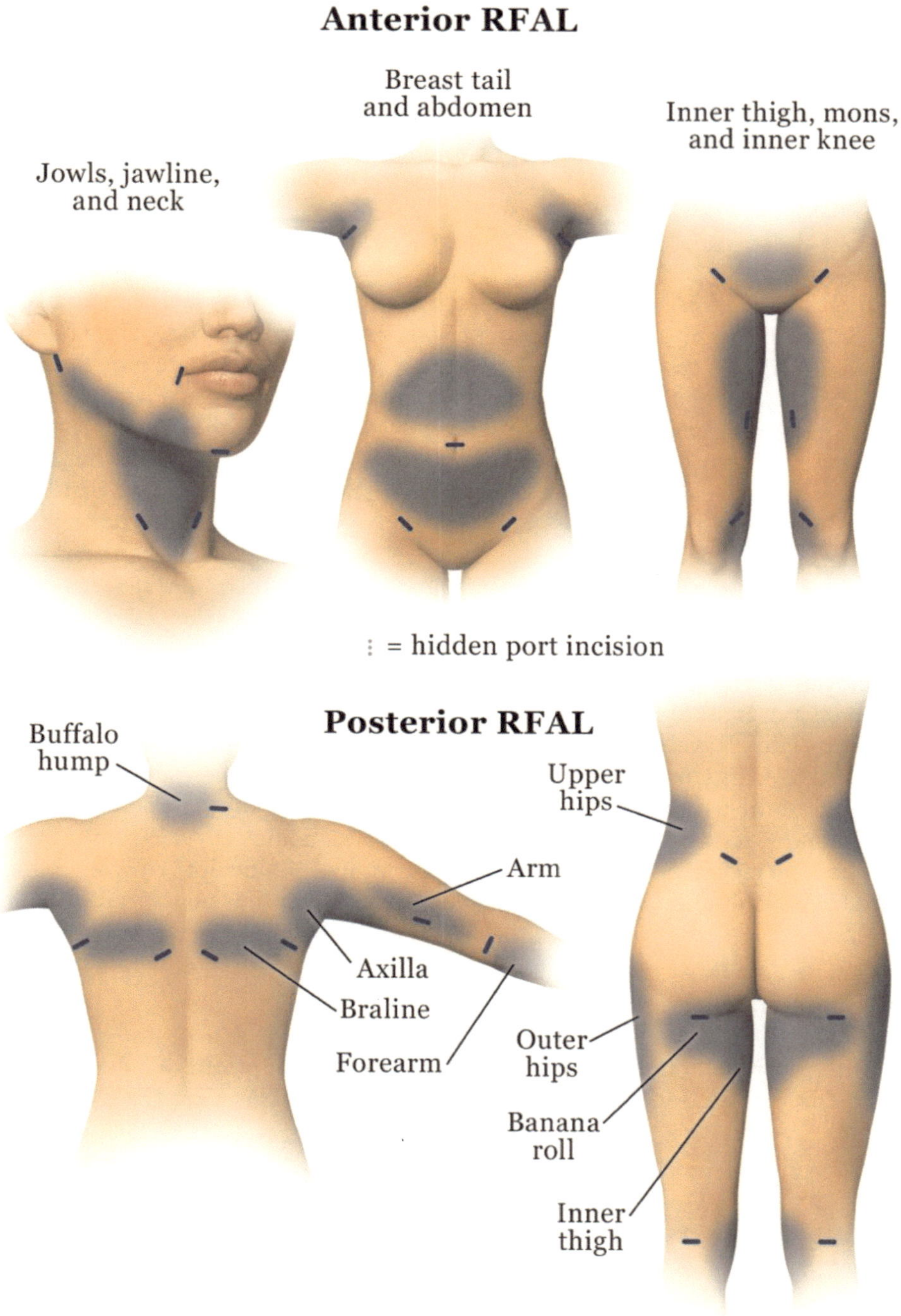

Figure 10.
Some of the standard BodyTite RFAL and aspiration ports.

device will deliver the precise amount of energy to heat the adipose at 20°C/cm³/s, while, for *International BodyTite®* users, the energy in watts will need to be entered and this will depend upon the hand piece selected and thickness of the flap. General energy settings for the international physicians are 50–60 W for the 3.7 mm × 25 cm and 17 cm large hand pieces, and 40–50 W for the 2.4 mm × 17 cm NeckTite® hand piece. For the FaceTite® 1.2 mm × 10 cm hand piece, 25 W is used. The New AccuTite® 0.9 mm × 8 cm applicator only requires 10–20 W.

3.6 Thermal end points

The thermal endpoints are thermal, 69–70° internal (USA) and 38–40° external cut off (USA and International). The final contour endpoints remain the art of the physician and are the aspiration endpoints.

3.7 Postoperative care

Postoperative BodyTite® care is similar to non-thermal liposuction and the author favors 6 weeks of compression garmenting. The first week is with silicone coated foam compression and the next 5 weeks the garment alone. For Abdominal RFAL BodyTite® cases, a small #7 JP drain is used, as seromas are much more common than with SAL, with an incidence approaching 8–10%. Presumably post RFAL seroma are more common resulting from temporary thermal damage of the lymphatics that takes some time to normalize. The drain is removed when there are three consecutive days with less than 20 cc of drainage each day. The first 3 weeks of garmenting are 22 h per day, which is reduced to 12 h a day (day or night time) for the next 3 weeks. Full ambulation is encouraged immediately, but return to low impact activities, such as an elliptical, stair climber, exercise bike at the end of 3 weeks and high impact exercise, running, spinning, etc. at the end of 6 weeks.

Noninvasive bulk heating devices, to achieve even better skin tightening can be deployed when the skin is less sensitive at 8–12 weeks. Shock wave devices can be used on any areas of lumps and areas of firmness.

BodyTite® leaves the skin very stiff, indurated and firmer for longer than non-thermal SAL/PAL or UAL and there is strong sense of tightness and contraction on the part of the patient for the first 6–9 months, which is the contraction process. At 3–6 months, for any areas of slight contour excess, noninvasive, localized fat destruction technologies, like SculpSure®, BodyFx®, EMSculpt®, CoolSculpting® and Ultrashape®, can be used to try to improve the contour non-surgically.

4. BodyTite®

Internationally there are 3 BodyTite® hand piece options, a 3.7 mm diameter × 25 cm or 17 cm long and a 2.4 mm × 17 cm long, also called the NeckTite®.

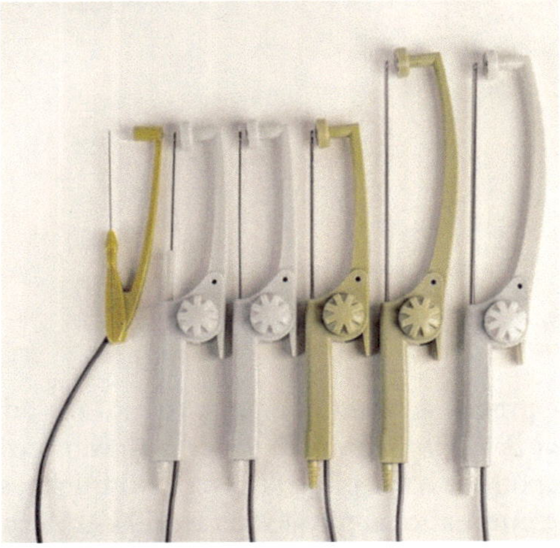

Figure 11.
The RFAL family of applicators, starting with the FaceTite® on the left, the BodyTite®/NeckTite® 2.4 mm, the CelluTite and the larger BodyTite® 3.7 mm × 25 cm (not all are available in the USA, but are internationally).

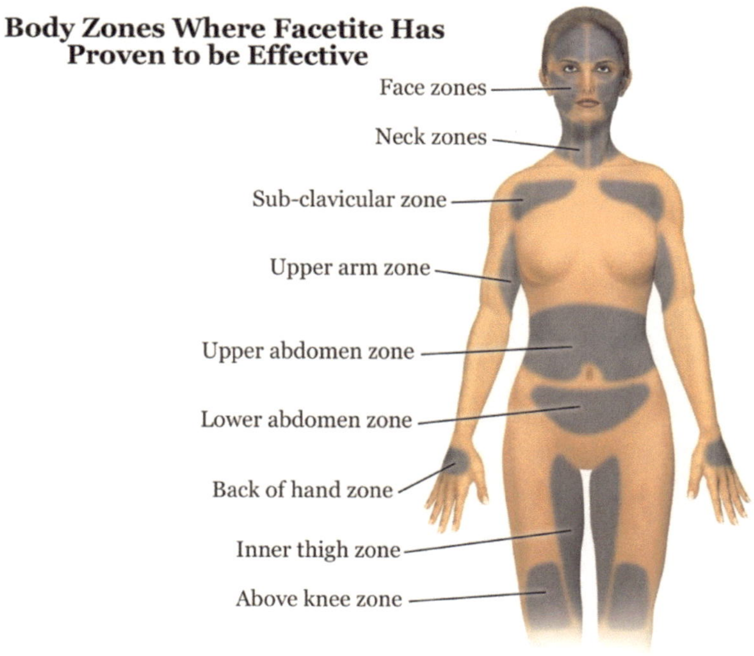

Figure 12.
Common areas where RFAL BodyTite®, FaceTite® and AccuTite® treatments can be effective.

The BodyTite® USA workstation comes in 20 W and 40 W configurations, the 40 W being more powerful and faster to endpoints and is called the BodyTite PRO (**Figure 11**). Both versions of the USA BodyTite® workstations automatically give as much power in watts as the treatment and hand piece needs to achieve the thermal velocity during the treatment of 20°C/cm^2/s and when this thermal velocity is exceeded (20–25°C/cm^2/s) will adjust down the energy until it is under 20°C/cm^3/s and if the rate of rise is >35°C/cm^2/s will shut off the energy flow and the foot pedal must be tapped again to being. The only BodyTite® hand piece currently available in the USA is the 2.4 mm × 17 cm hand piece.

Following the protocols and parameters outlined above, excellent results using RFAL thermal coagulation can be achieved. The areas that may benefit from BodyTite® and RFAL are outline in **Figures 12, 13**.

5. NeckTite (BodyTite 2.4 mm)

The NeckTite® is available internationally and is 2.4 mm × 17 cm and was originally designed for large necks, but has become the smaller BodyTite hand piece for smaller adipose zones in the non USA markets, while the 3.7 mm diameter hand piece is used for the larger body zones. With the introduction of the FaceTite Internationally and in the USA, the FaceTite(R) has become the RFAL applicator used most commonly for jawline, necks and very small body zones.

For International physicians, the external electrode of the 2.4 mm × 17 cm NeckTite® hand piece is much smaller in diameter than the BodyTite® 3.7 mm external electrode and, as such, has a much higher power density, is more efficient and heats tissue much more quickly and with less energy.

Using the protocol and parameters outlined above, excellent small zone Body contouring results can be achieved with the 2.4 mm × 17 cm hand piece and is most commonly used on the inner thighs, bra line, arms and smaller abdominal convexities (**Figure 12**).

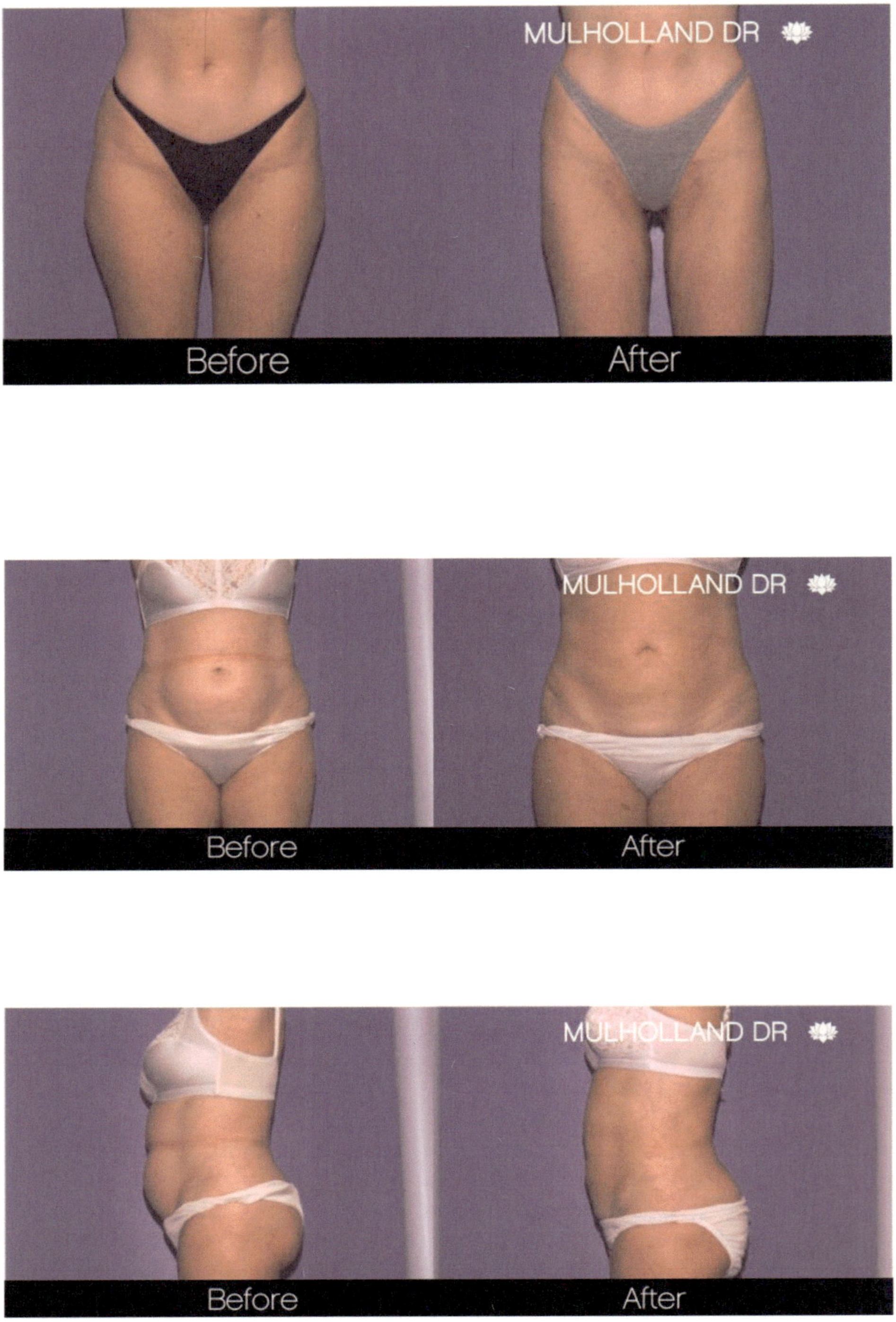

Figure 13.
BodyTite® before and after result at 12 months. Top panel RFAL was performed on the inner and outer tight of a 45-year-old and the middle and bottom panel BodyTite® was performed on the abdomen and hips in 68-year-old patient.

6. FaceTite

The FaceTite® is a very small RFAL applicator, designed for the neck, jawline, face and very small body contouring areas and is great for small secondary liposuction enhancements where fibrofatty tissue, which is like cement, can be anticipated (**Figures 14**, **15**).

In both the USA and Internationally, the FaceTite® hand piece is 1.2 mm in diameter × 10 cm long and is a solid, non-aspirating electrode (even internationally). The distance between the internal and external electrode is controlled by pinching the electrodes together to create the desired interelectrode distance, rather than a fixed dial, prior to entering the subcutaneous fat. Again, super-wet tumescent fluid is infiltrated prior to treatment (**Figure 15**).

Using the protocols and parameters listed below, excellent results can be achieved tightening along the jawline and neck and small body contouring areas. The treatment of the jawline, submentum and neck can be performed using a three port approach, with a single submental port accessing the submentum and neck for

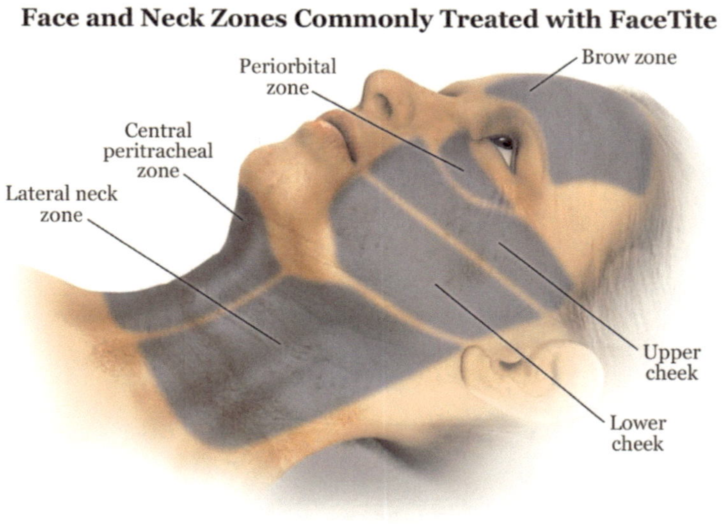

Figure 14.
Areas of the face and neck that can be treated with the FaceTite® and AccuTite®.

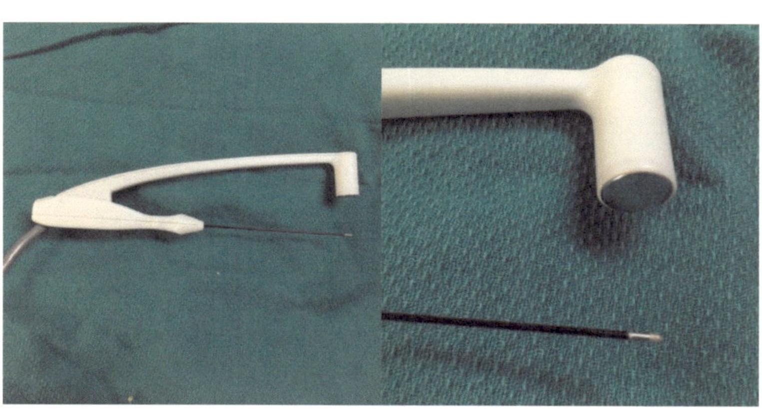

Figure 15.
The FaceTite® applicator.

RFAL and aspiration. Two more lateral ports are used to thermocoagulate and tighten each jowls and jawline. These Jawline and jowl ports can be either at the inferior border of the mandible at the lateral aspects of the submental crease on either side, or, through a sub-lobular port (**Figure 16**).

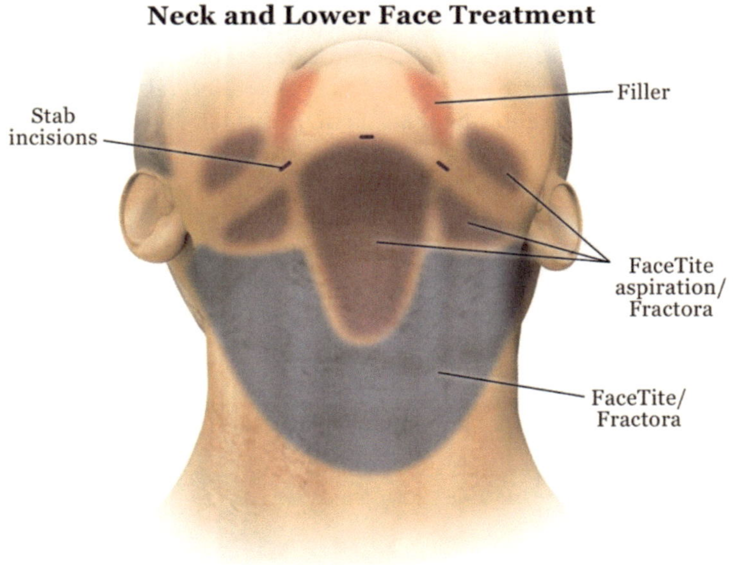

Figure 16.
The FaceTite® RFAL approach to the submentum, neck and jawline.

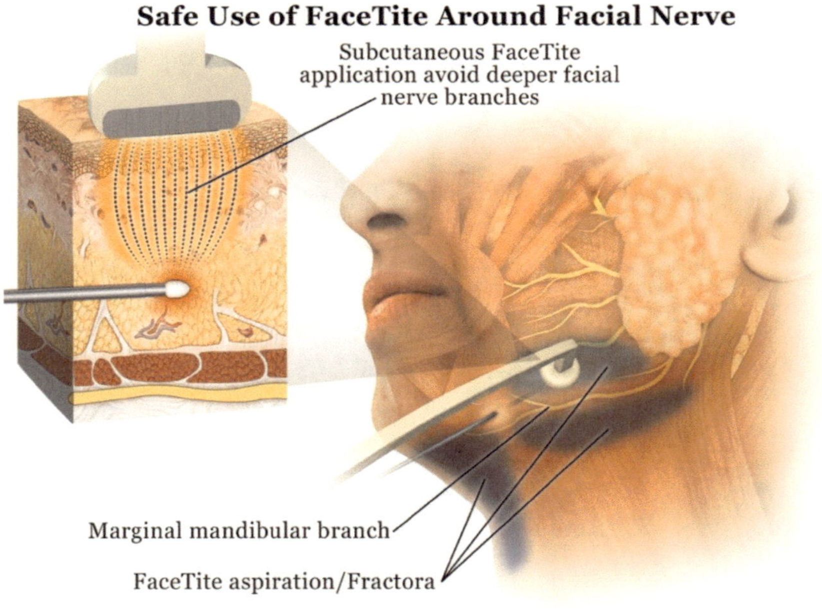

Figure 17.
Keep the internal electrode of the FaceTite® above the SMAS and platysma, working in the very superficial fat, to protect injury to the marginal mandibular branch of the facial nerve.

When working over the jawline, the FaceTite® physician must ensure that the internal electrode is above the SMAS and platysma, in the subcutaneous space to minimize the risk to the facial nerve. Because the RF flow is from the internal

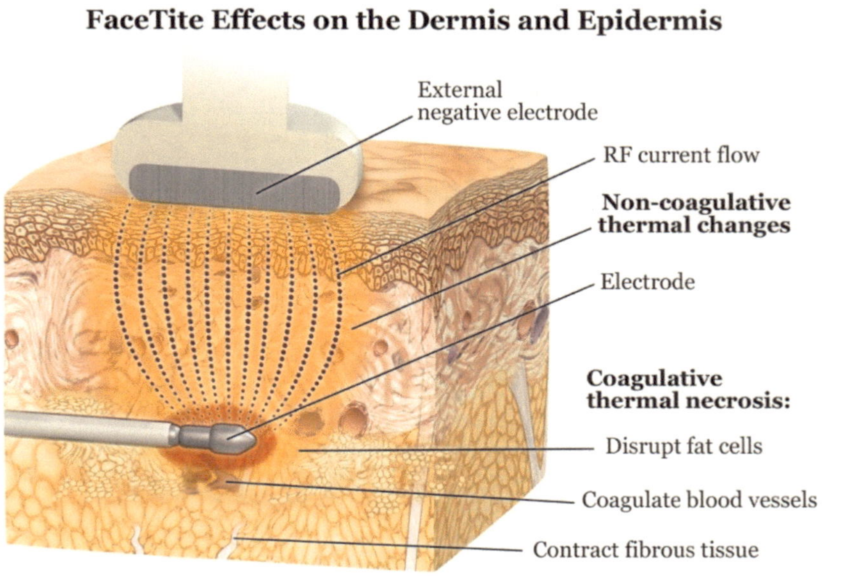

Figure 18.
For skin tightening and contraction, the FaceTite is passed with the superficial fat just under the dermis. Always leave 3–6 mm of fat between the internal electrode and the dermis. Adipose coagulation and dermal remodeling lead to tightening of the skin. Aspiration may or may not be performed depending upon the area.

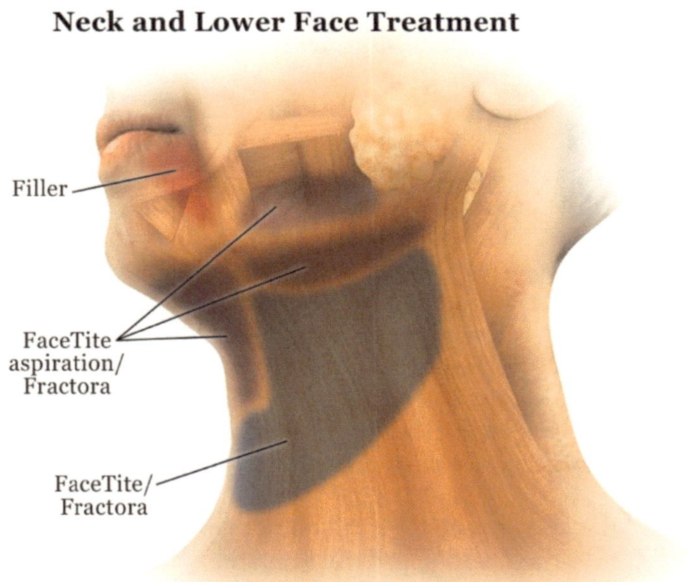

Figure 19.
The FaceTite® can be used superficially to deliver skin tightening without aspiration (jawline) or within the jowl, submental and neck fat and modest aspiration performed after for contour.

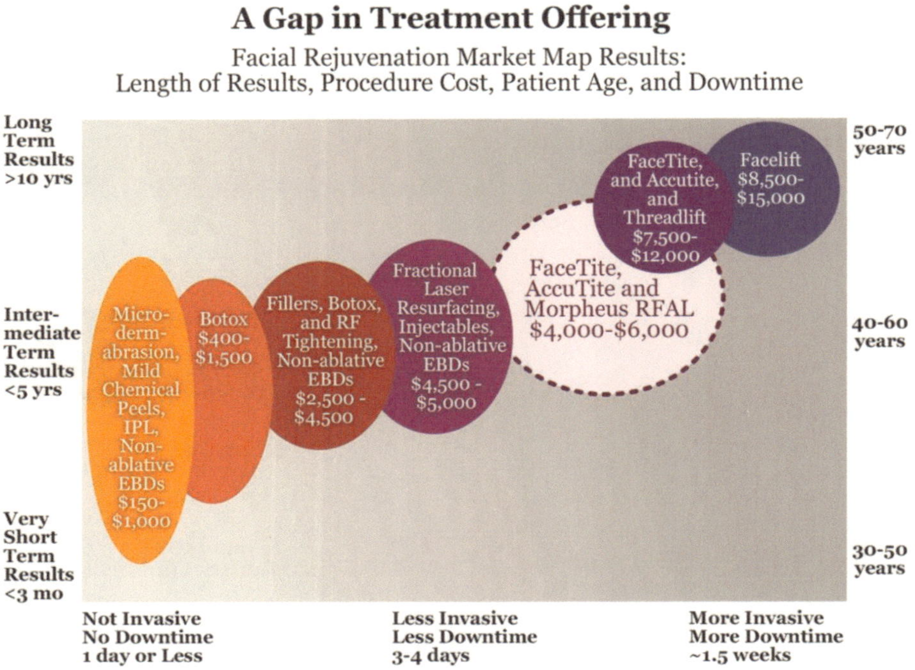

Figure 20.
The FaceTite® and AccuTite® can fill the gap in therapeutic options between more aggressive excisional procedures, like a facelift and the completely noninvasive external energy-based device (EBD) treatments and injectables.

electrode up to the external electrode, there is a "thermal containment" which is not present in other mono-probe systems, minimizing a thermal neuropraxia of the marginal mandibular branch of the facial nerve (**Figure 17**).

When performing RFAL along the jawline, the FaceTite RFAL lipocoagulation is executed using a slow moving and/or stamping technique within the superficial fat, just under the dermis (**Figure 18**). Always leave 3–5 mm of fat between the internal electrode and the dermis. The thermal endpoints are 69° in the superficial fat (US systems), a popping sound (International) and a skin cut off temperature of 38–40°. The FaceTite® can be performed just under the skin of the jawline and jowl to create significant skin tightening and firming of the jawline with reduction of the Jowl. Minimal or even no suction may be used in this region.

When using the FaceTite in the submentum and neck, the internal electrode is passed through the submental fat pad, coagulating the adipose and delivering soft tissue contraction with deep endpoints being 69° (USA) or popping (International) and the skin temperature is brought to 38–40° (**Figure 19**). In the submentum and neck, suction aspiration is performed after the heating if there is a fatty deposit.

The FaceTite® and the newer AccuTite® can provide the liposuction surgeon with a procedure that "bridges the gap" between non-invasive face and skin tightening and the more invasive excisional procedures like a facelift (**Figures 20, 21**).

The FaceTite ®can also be used for small, focal liposuction body zones with little fat, to ensure soft tissue contraction prior to aspiration. Zones such as the upper arms, inner thighs, upper abdomen, as well as the jawline and neck as easily treated with the FaceTite®.

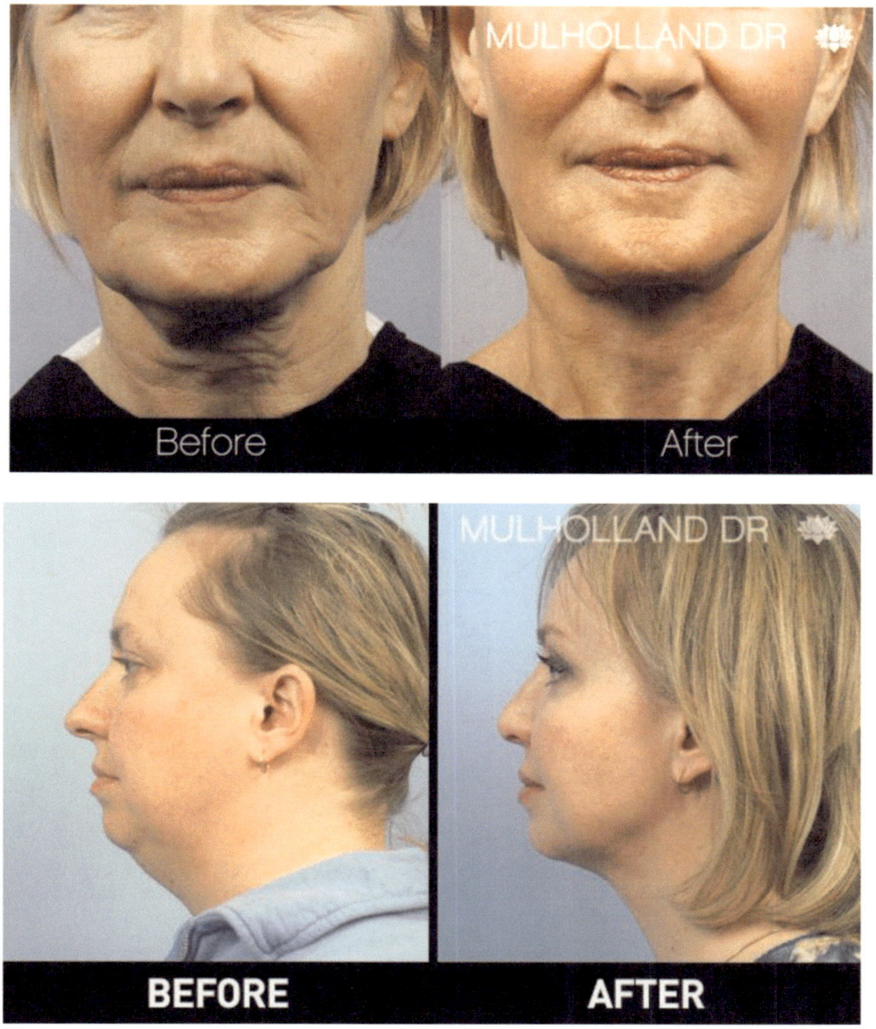

Figure 21.
Top panel is FaceTite® of the jawline and jowl, with FaceTite® and Morpheus of the neck. Bottom panel is FaceTite® and liposuction of the submentum and neck.

7. CelluTite

The CelluTite hand piece has a V-dissector shape plastic tip, rather than bullet shaped and is used to treat advanced, grade 3 nodulo-pitted cellulite of the buttock and thighs. The hand piece is 2.4 mm × 17 cm long (**Figure 22**).

The CelluTite® is designed to treat the three anatomic pathologies of Cellulite

i. nodules,

ii. pits, and

iii. dermal thinning with adipose herniation.

Cellulite patients tend to have a more vertically oriented FSN anatomy and, over many years there is a contraction of many of the vertically oriented fibroseptal bands and edema of the superficial fat which leads to the pits and nodules characteristic of more advance cellulite (**Figure 23**).

The CelluTite® patient is marked out in the standing position and all deep pits are marked for release, while the nodules are marked using a different color and are targeted for stamping and popping to reduce the nodules. The thinned dermis, that allows superficial fat herniation is then heated, thickened and minimizes the ability of superficial fat to herniate into the dermis.

Only superficial tumescent anesthesia is required (first 4–6 cm of soft tissue) and a tense tumescent infiltration is instilled. The entire treatment is performed at level 2 on the CelluTite® depth setting. The procedure is divided into releasing the

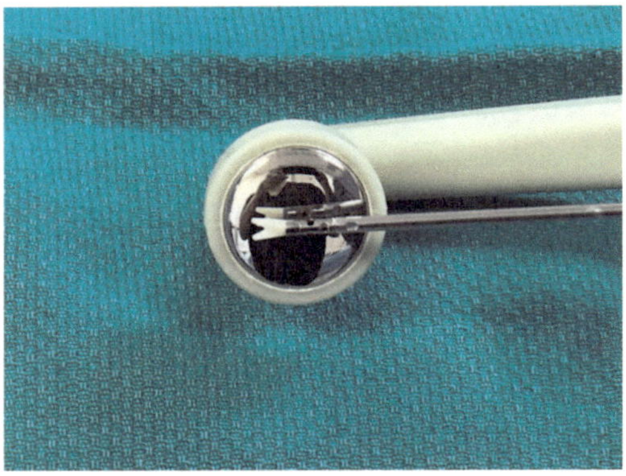

Figure 22.
The CelluTite® has a V-shaped tip, making the CelluTite® a thermal V dissector. The V-tip, traps the vertical, shortened, fibroseptal band that pulls down the dermis causing the deep skin pits. The band undergoes a thermolysis, release the pit and smoothening the skin.

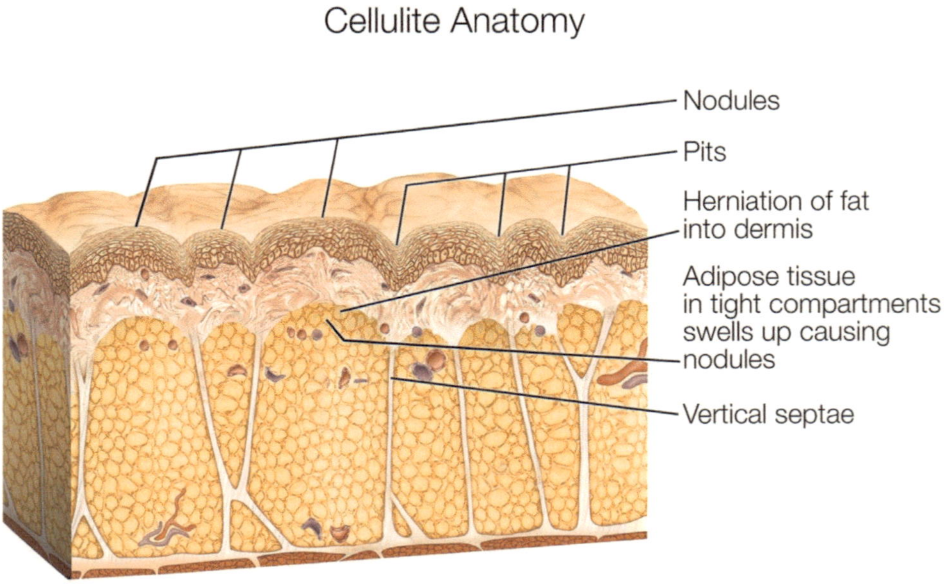

Figure 23.
The anatomy of cellulite: the FSN tends to be more vertically oriented. The pits are caused by shortened fibroseptal bands. Nodules result from edematous, swelling of superficial fat from the microcirculatory compromise. The dermis is thin, leading to fat herniating into the reticular dermis.

pits, followed by coagulation and reduction of the nodules. To release the pits, CelluTite tip is advanced the slowly at several levels across each pit. The thermal V-dissector captures the contracted FSN which is causing the dimple at the apex of the V (**Figure 24**) and bends the FSN over the RF emitting internal electrode, result in a thermoseptolysis and release, which allows the pitted skin to "pop back up" and smoothen the pitted appearance to the skin.

Additional smoothening is then achieved by moving the internal electrode up under a pre-marked nodule and performing a stationary stamping technique under each nodule and heating until the cutoff of 69° is achieved (USA) or, for International physicians, for 2 s, until there is a "popping" sound, both of which coagulate the edematous herniated fat, flattening the area and smoothening the contour (**Figure 25**).

Once all the pits and nodules have been successful performed, slow back and forth passes are made under the soft tissue until there is no FSN resistance with each pass and the external skin temperature reaches the pre-set cut off of 38–40°C. This will provide additional dermal thickening, minimizing herniated dermal fat (**Figure 26**).

Excellent long term CelluTite® results can be achieved with a single treatment, often 50–70% reduction (**Figure 27**) which can last for many years (22). Recurrent nodulo-pitted irregularity is prevented by the creation of more multi-directional FSN, than the vertically oriented anatomy that contributed to the deformity and this multi-directional, remodeled FSN is resistant to any single fibroseptal band to shortening and causing a deep pit (**Figure 28**).

CelluTite® can be performed at the same time as BodyTite® and aspiration liposuction. Generally, in combination cases, CelluTite® of the buttock, posteriorly

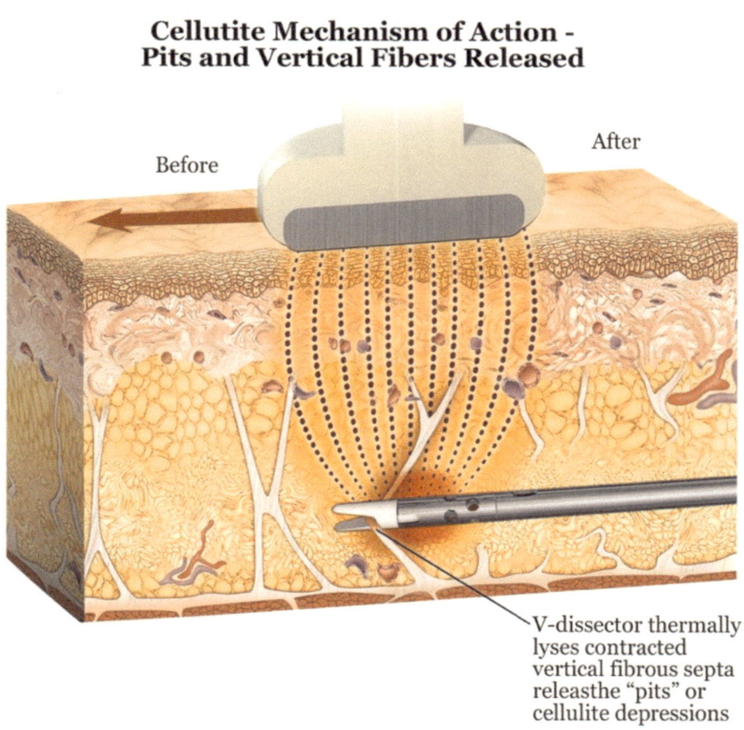

Figure 24.
The thermal V dissector captures the shortened vertical fibroseptal band(s) in the apex of the V and bends the band over the thermal electrode causing a thermoseptolysis and band division. This slow back and forth release is repeated a several vertical depth, providing a thorough release. This allows the pitted skin to "pop' back up smoothening the overlying skin.

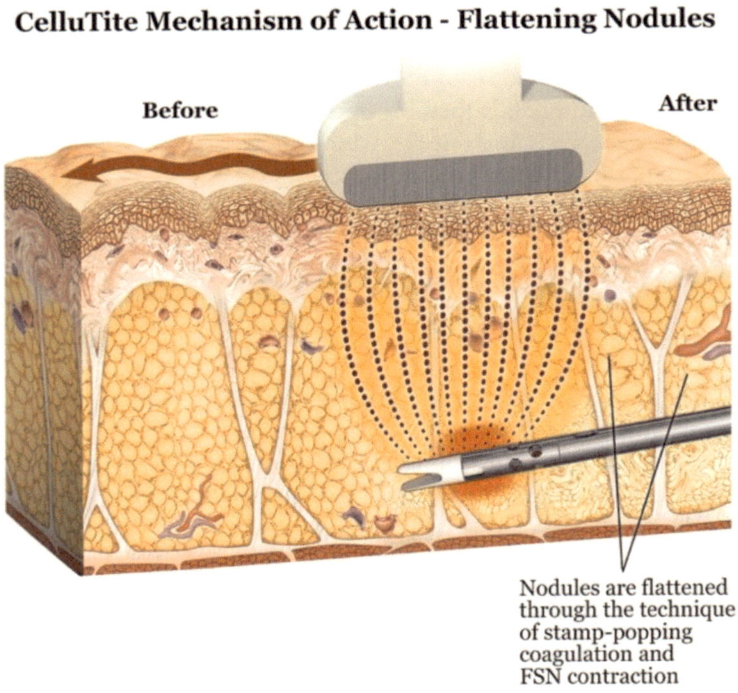

Figure 25.
The CelluTite® applicator is placed under a nodule and a stationary stamping technique is performed causing coagulation of the nodule (70° cut off in the USA BodyTite® platforms and popping after 2 s in international BodyTite® systems). This coagulates the edematous fat and flattens the nodular skin.

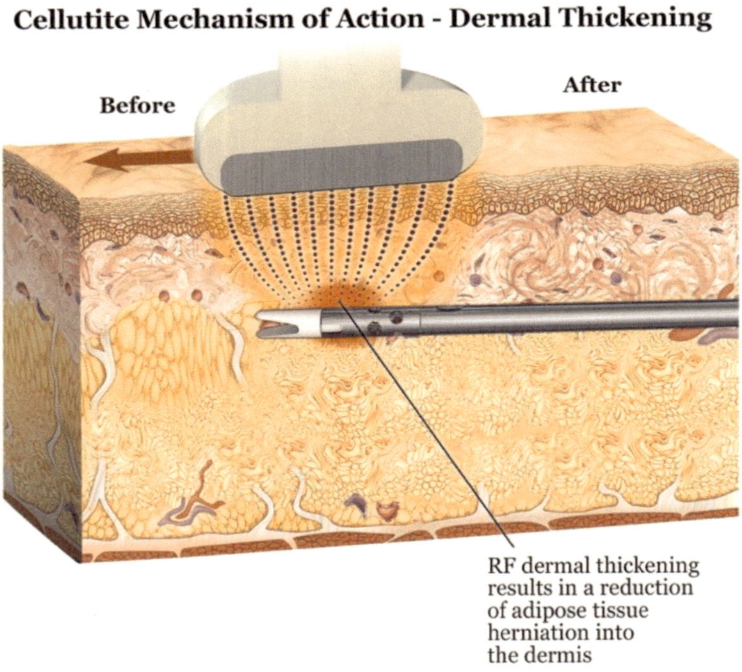

Figure 26.
The skin and dermis are then heated to 38–40°C superficially and the subdermal space to 69° (US systems), thickening the dermis and reducing fat herniating into the dermis.

and laterally is performed superficially first, follow immediately by BodyTite® RFAL liposuction of the outer and inner thighs second.

Non-invasive suction coupled RF devices such as the BodyFX®, Velashap. 3®, Venus Legacy® and others can be used after 6 weeks of garmenting to maintain the outcome and protect the patient's improvement.

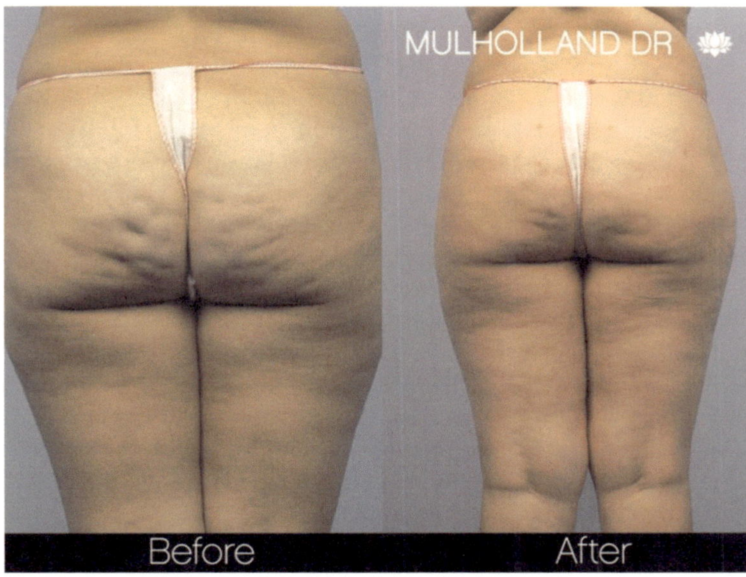

Figure 27.
Long term, 36 month results of CelluTite of the buttock.

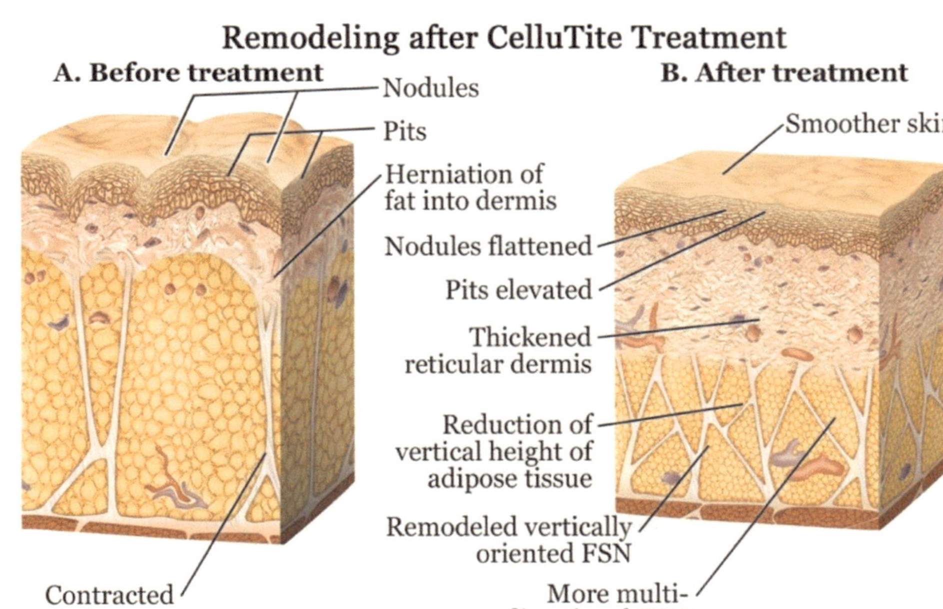

Figure 28.
With release of the pits, flattening of the nodules and thickening of the skin, the remodeling process leads to a more multi-directional FSN network, which is resistant to shortening of individual bands and nodular swelling of the fat.

8. AccuTite®: injectable RF and skin tightening

The AccuTite® is the newest and smallest of the BodyTite® RFAL applicators and can be deployed on any of the BodyTite® workstations (the 20 W and the 40 W BodyTite® Pro as well as the new Embrace RF workstation). The AccuTite® has all the thermal, impedance and contact automated monitoring and feedback as the BodyTite®, FaceTite® and CelluTite® applicators, but it is very versatile by nature of its tiny size. The internal solid, silicone coated electrode is only 0.9 mm in diameter and is 8 cm long. The entire Bipolar RFAL applicator can fit easily into the palm of your hand (**Figures 29, 30**). The AccuTite® is smaller than most of the conventional microcannulas being used to inject soft tissue fillers in the deep subcutaneous and supra-periosteal space (**Figures 29, 30**). The AccuTite® appeals to virtually every physician, both the surgeon and non-surgeon users who are looking for safe, predictable, non-excisional methods of coagulating fat and tightening skin. Physician users can think of AccuTite® as *Injectable RF and Injectable skin tightening.*

The small size of the AccuTite® allows the physician us use a small #21-gauge port creation needle anywhere on the face, neck and body where skin needs to be tightened, with or without lipoaspiration. Once under the skin, the stamping and moving techniques for thermal coagulation are deployed, with the cut off temperatures of 69° internal and 38–40° external being deployed. When used subdermally for skin tightening, no aspiration is required.

The AccuTite® can be used to coagulate fat and tighten the FSN prior to liposuction and aspiration in very small zones. The #21-gauge port needle site need not be closed with a suture and the physician can simply "pop in and out" of lax skin zones all over the body, including the upper and lower lid and perioral, jawline and neck (**Figure 31**).

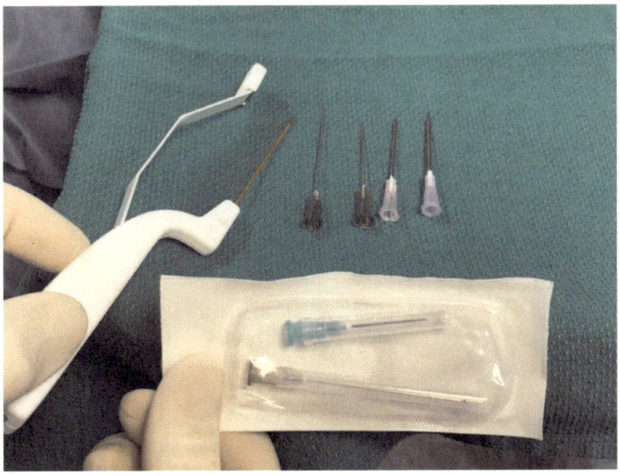

Figure 29.
The AccuTite® is the smallest of the RFAL hand pieces. It is 0.9 mm in diameter and can fit into the palm of your hand. The internal electrode is inserted under the skin to remodel the deep reticular dermis to 70°, while the external electrode will move along the surface of the skin and heat to 40–42°. The AccuTite® is shown above, next to a commonly used 22 gauge microcannula and the internal AccuTite® electrode is actually smaller. A 21-gauge needle is used to create an insertion port for the AccuTite®, which is then inserted under the skin and RF is injected under the dermis, resulting in skin and soft tissue tightening, hence, the ***term injectable RF.***

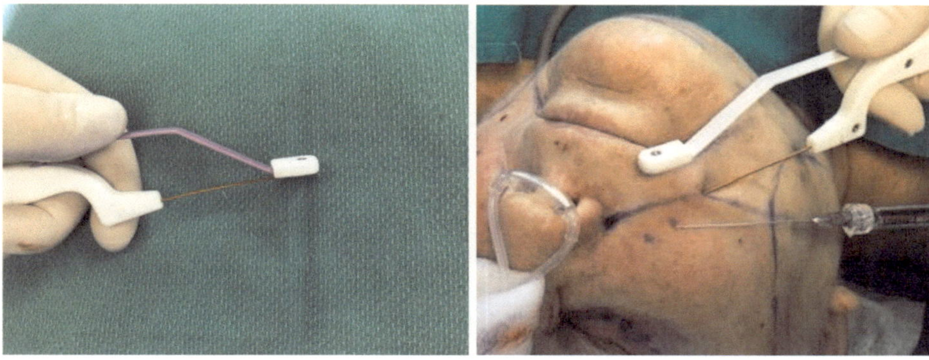

Figure 30.
The AccuTite ®is small and easy to control. Above it is being used to tighten the para-nasiolabial smile line tissue and, following that, Juvederm is being injected through the same plane at a deeper level. The AccuTite® can be used under local anesthesia together with your soft tissue fillers and at the same time, often using many of the same tactics and skill sets.

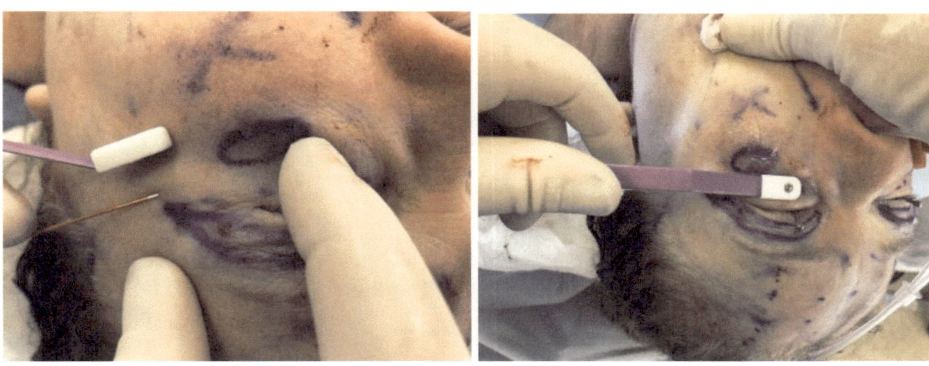

Figure 31.
The small, compact size of AccuTite® and the small size of the internal and external electrode, allows this versatile RFAL applicator to gain access to areas of loose skin all over the face, neck and body. Despite its small size, the sub-dermal space is heated quickly and effectively to the same thermal endpoints as are used by BodyTite ® and FaceTite®, with the thermal endpoint of the subdermal space being 70° and the skin cut-off of 40°C. Skin tightening is significant and the small port access means a suture is not even needed for an access port.

9. Morpheus: external RFAL

The Morpheus is an externally applied fractional radiofrequency assisted lipocoagulation (RFAL) device that has been developed to help tighten and contract soft tissue, and contour superficial fat and skin texture at the time of liposuction, or as a stand-alone procedure. For the liposuction surgeon, once the BodyTite®, FaceTite®, AccuTite® or CelluTite® device has been deployed and the aspiration of the fat completed, a final step of lipocoagulation can be performed using the Morpheus, from *"outside the skin in"*. The Morpheus is an external applicator, loaded on the BodyTite® and Embrace RF workstations that delivers 24 silicone coated pins into the superficial, subdermal layers of the fat. Think of each pin-triangular exit point as a tiny BodyTite electrode system. Each pin is 300 microns in diameter, has an uncoated tip and is positively charged. The physician can control the depth of the pin extrusion and a 100 ms RF pulse of positively charged current is emitted upon

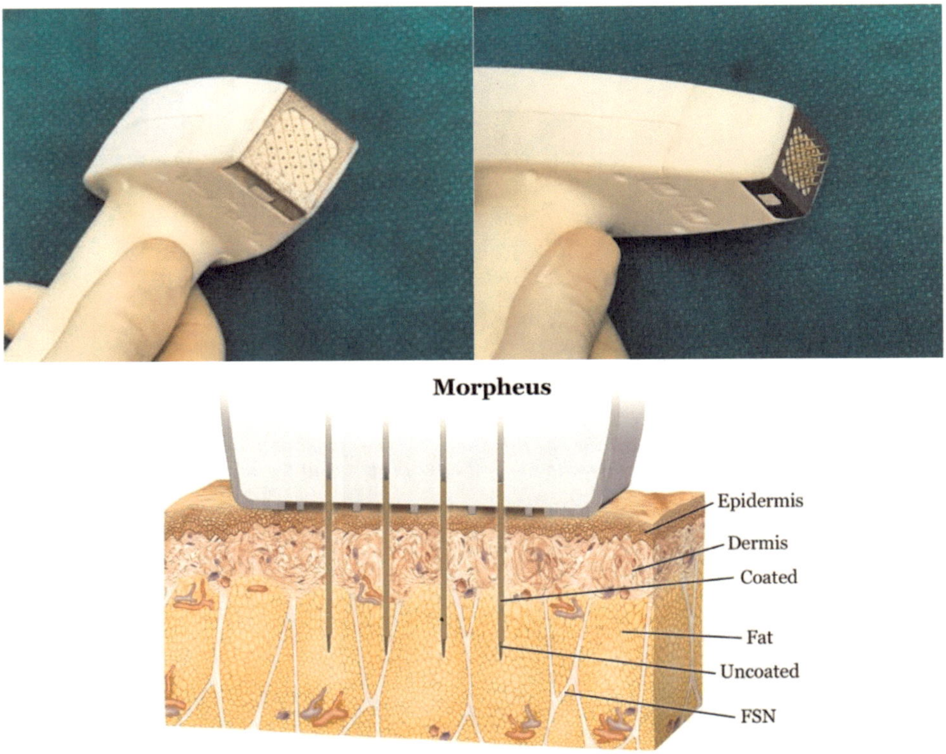

Figure 32.
The Morpheus is an external applied micro bipolar RFAL device, that emits a 24 pin, positively charged array into the adipose tissue under the skin. Each needle, like RFAL, is a positively charged electrode that penetrates the fat and then releases ablative RF energy that flows up to a negative electrode on top of the skin.

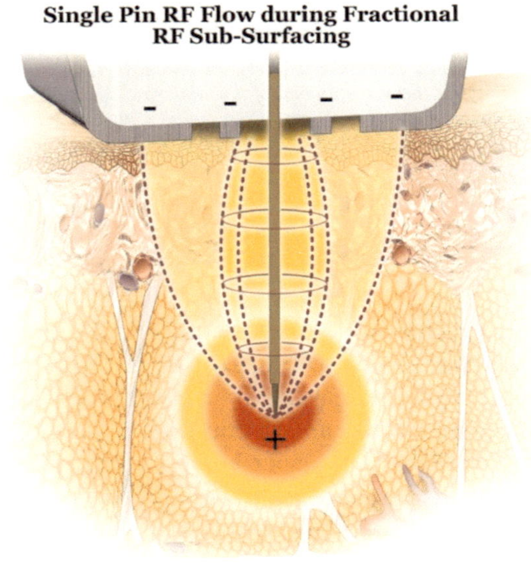

Figure 33.
The tiny, coated, positive charged electrodes are inserted into the superficial fat, and, when the RF energy is released, a zone of ablation and adipose coagulation is created with each pulse, leading to FSN contraction and soft tissue contouring and tightening. The RF flows up to the negatively charged triangular shaped electrodes which creates a strong, non-ablative dermal remodeling effect of the each of the.

maximal extrusion. The triangular shaped exit point of the pin, is negatively charged and acts as the primary return electrode for the flow of RF from the tip of the pin, created a bipolar lipocoagulation system similar to BodyTite® (**Figure 32**).

Like BodyTite®, the Morpheus emits RF energy is ablative and coagulative near the uncoated tip of the pin and then, the RF energy flows strongly up the coated pin to a triangular shaped negative electrode. The RF pulse creates a zone of ablation several hundred microns in diameter that coagulates the fat and tightens the FSN (**Figures 33, 34**). The RF current then flows up the pin to the negatively charged, triangular electrodes located at pin exit sites on the tip to provide a bipolar, non-ablative thermal stimulation effect on the reticular and papillary dermis (**Figures 33, 34**). RF also flows form the positively charged, mono polar pin tip to the widely space negatively charge rails on the sides of the tip for a gentle sub-necrotic heating and the entire zone (**Figures 33, 34**).

Basically, each of the 24 needles acts like a mini-BodyTite® internal electrode. Because the needle is silicon coated, there is no thermal epidermal-dermal effect

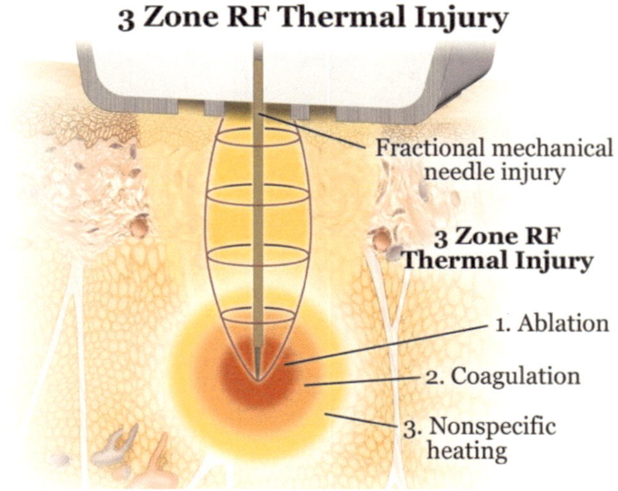

Figure 34.
The zone of ablation and adipose coagulation contracts the FSN and contracts the soft tissue. The flow of RF up to the negative electrodes creates a more gentler, sub-necrotic, non-ablative heating and tightening of the dermis.

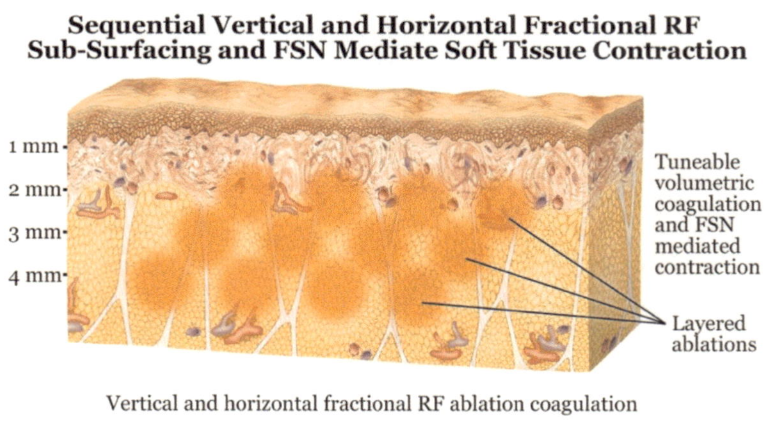

Figure 35.
Multiple pass and variable depth Morpheus will lead to vertical sequential FSN contraction, contouring and skin tightening.

and the ablation occurs around the positively charted, uncoated tip and is within the superficial fat using the FSN as the main vehicle for soft tissue contouring and tightening (**Figures 33, 34**).

The physician can set the pin penetration depth to periocular (approx. 2 mm), face (3 mm) and body (4 mm) and treat at multiple sequential depths to create a vertical and horizontal fractional thermal stimulation and optimal contraction. The Morpheus is an excellent final step in BodyTite®, FaceTite®, AccuTite® and CelluTite® treatment to obtain superficial liporeduction, lipocoagulation and soft tissue tightening.

Like with BodyTite®, multiple passes of the Morpheus will allow the physician to create a vertical thermal lipocoagulation with skin tightening and remodeling. This horizontal and vertical thermal lipocoagulation leads to excellent skin tightening and can be done in contraction (**Figure 35, 36**).

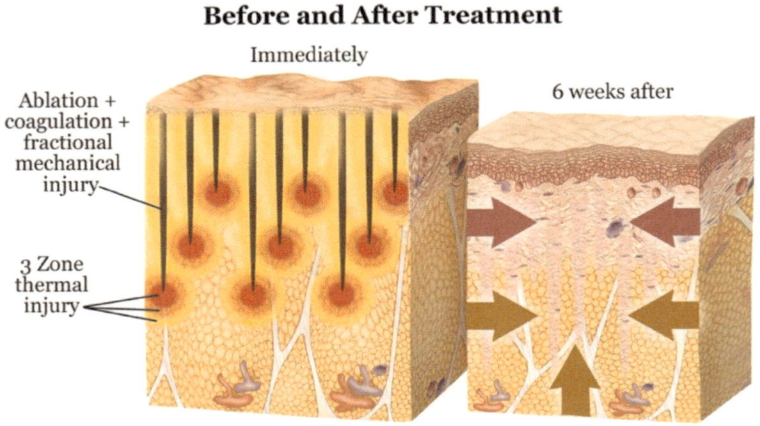

Figure 36.
Multiple pass, sequential vertical and horizontal Morpheus RFAL will lead to 3D soft tissue contraction and tightening.

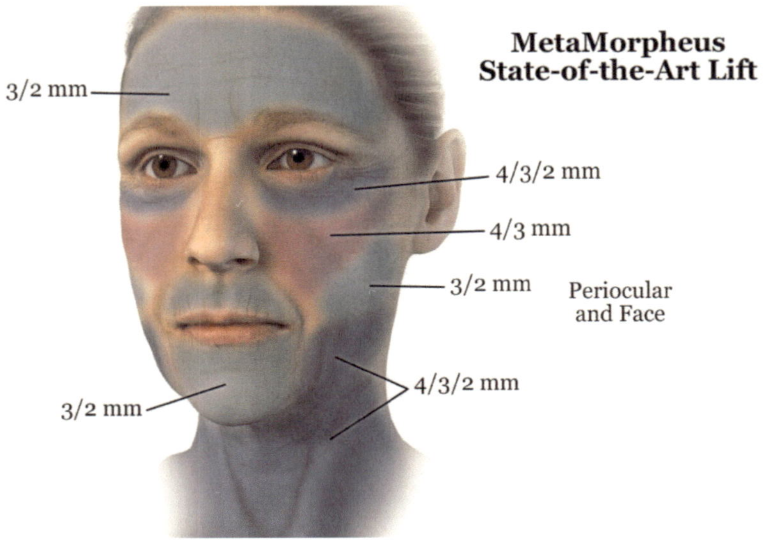

Figure 37.
The Morpheus can afford the liposuction surgeon, an external mini RFAL device that delivers 24 tiny mini BodyTite RFAL thermal injury injuries and can result in significant skin contraction. This can provide a nonexcisional face and necklift like result.

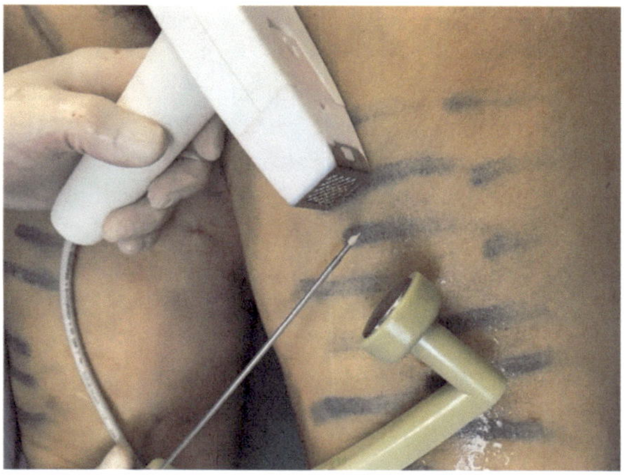

Figure 38.
CelluTite® or BodyTite®, FaceTite® and AccuTite® can be combined with Morpheus to enhance the overall soft tissue contraction and skin tightening with an "inside out" and "outside in" thermal sandwich approach.

The Morpheus can be offered on the face, or body, and after a treatment with a BodyTite® liposuction procedure for enhanced contraction and skin tightening after liposuction (**Figures 36**, **37**).

When Morpheus is used on the face, multiple pass, multiple depth approach is used. The deep pass is ablative and coagulative in the deep layer, often the frontalis, orbicularis, SMAS and platysmal. The next pass coagulated the subdermal fat and the final pass into the fat of the subdermal space (**Figure 37**).

The Morpheus can be combined with BodyTite RFAL liposuction to improve overall soft tissue contraction and skin tightening (**Figure 38**).

10. Combination excision and RFAL

The ability to achieve significant BodyTite® RFAL contraction has opened a more minimal excisional opportunity for surgeons in achieving optimal contouring results with less invasive procedures. Mini intra-pubic skin pinch tummy tucks, removing infra-umbilical skin excess with BodyTite® RFAL upper and lower abdominal lipocoagulation and aspiration can achieve results of a full abdominoplasty, with less scarring when the rectus abdominus diastasis is not significant. Axillary mini-brachioplasty with BodyTite® lipocoagulation and aspiration of the arm, limited incision, inguinal Anterior thigh lifting with BodyTite® liposuction to the inner thigh and lateral post or periauricular lateral face and neck-lifting with anterior compartment FaceTite® RFAL and lipoaspiration are all examples of combining BodyTite® RFAL applicators in combination with more minimal excisional approaches to achieve excellent results in selected patients.

By combining the contraction power of RFAL with more minimal limited excisional approach, a less invasive option between totally non excisional energy based device treatments and full excisional, more standard lifting is created that gives patients the option for a better outcome than an EBD without the excisional scars, or recovery of a typical open surgery. Often these BodyTite® assisted procedures can be performed as an outpatient, under oral and tumescent anesthesia and nitrous oxide inhalational, avoiding a full general anesthetic. This BodyTite® RFAL together with the mini-lift, give physician an *"in between"* option that is more appealing to patients and can give a superior outcome with less scarring or downtime.

11. BodyTite® RFAL and other liposuction technologies

BodyTite® RFAL is an industry leading lipocoagulation skin tightening technology and technique, with documented 35% soft tissue and skin area contraction. The physician still needs to perform final aspiration and contouring. Small, microcannula SAL, PAL (MicroAire, Vaser PAL or Tickle Lipo) are the most common aspiration options. UAL, Ultrasound assisted may be deployed prior to BodyTite®, particularly if fat grafting is being performed, as UAL will facilitate fat cell decohesion, separation and then aspiration and collection of the adipose tissue, BUT these adipocytes and adipocyte derived stem cells *will be viable* and survive the fat grafting process.

SmartLipo®, or laser assisted liposuction (LAL) is another viable thermocoagulation soft tissue tightening system, with documented 17% area contraction. LAL is not as efficient as RFAL with inferior published skin contraction data, but, is a very strong brand and can be easily marketed. Occasionally, the physicians with both SmartLipo® and BodyTite®, may use the laser lipolysis for a small, and often subdermal component of the procedure and then deploy the BodyTite® applicator for the majority of the thermal coagulation process. Propulsive water assisted liposuction (WAL), is gentle, with less bruising, but does not lead to enhanced soft tissue contraction, so is not a common technology in most regions of the world. Plasma assisted liposuction is relatively new and can deliver soft tissue contraction, but lacks internal thermal control, is relatively slow and plasma may be better suited and relegated to external skin resurfacing.

BodyTite® is usually the stand along soft tissue contraction system and can be performed before the final aspiration contouring or, after aspiration and contouring has been performed. There are no studies confirming which, RFAL before or after aspiration, delivers the best contraction and results. The author does prefer to perform BodyTite® RFAL first, not just to optimize the number of FSN architecture that can be shortened prior to aspiration, BUT, also to ensure, small venule and arterioles undergo a thermal coagulation and then, when aspiration is performed last, there is less injury and bleeding into the subcutaneous space with less patient ecchymosis. The coagulation and liquification of fat, means more gentle aspiration forces are required, which likely translates into less edema, swelling and pain.

12. RFAL complications

The use of body tight RFAL applicators has evolved into a very safe and efficacious tool. Over 10,000 procedures have been performed worldwide with a very low complication rate. However, like any surgical tool untoward outcomes can occur and the risk of complication is often proportionate to the therapeutic index of safety of the device and the experience of the surgeon. Fortunately, over the past 10 years of BodyTite® innovation in the thermal lipocoagulation, there has been a tremendous evolution in the onboard sensing of soft tissue thermal profiles and automated modulation of the radiofrequency output around those variables.

12.1 Thermal injury

Contact sensor, high and low impedance sensors, external and internal electrothermal cutoffs, audible warnings as temperature rises, automated cut off

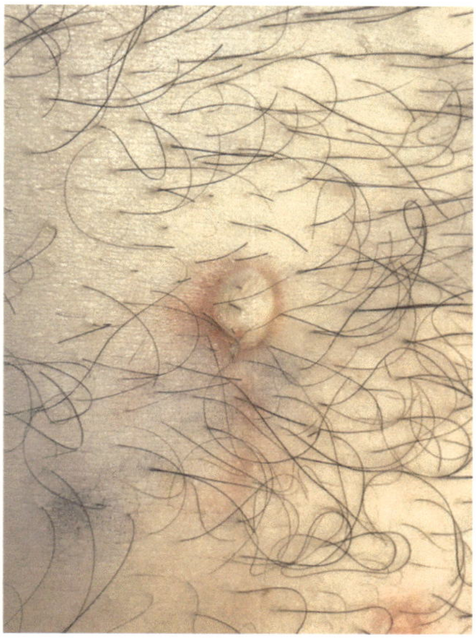

Figure 39.
A small full thickness BodyTite® burn during abdominal RFAL treatment. Secondary intent healing and remodeling, with dilute triamcinolone (Kenalog 2) injections will result is a very cosmetically acceptable result.

temperatures, and energy output linked to the rate of rise of temperature with temperature surge protection are all part of myriad of onboard thermal control systems. Despite these safety features there is a small risk of a thermal injury. Because the heating from the subcutaneous level up through the, any thermal excess, any thermal excess will result in a full thickness burn. The vast majority these thermal injuries are small and limited nature and heal by secondary intent and occasional required excision once the scar has softened and remodeled (**Figure 39**).

This risk a thermal injury far less than 0.25% (1 in 400 cases) and diminishes with the experience of the physician. To minimize the risk of a burner thermal injury conservative settings and parameters as outlined in this chapter and advanced training environments and experience, together with an adequate amount of tumescent anesthesia, and avoid peri-port injuries will make out the risk of the thermal excess very uncommon. When a peri-port burn occurs in a esthetically sensitive region, like the face or neck, the author will perform an epidermal closure over the injury, rather allow secondary intent healing and perform fractional RF or CO_2 treatment once this is healed or, perform a secondary scar revision if necessary (**Figure 40**).

12.2 Nodules

In the past BodyTite® and its RFL applicators lacked the sophisticated internal thermal monitoring and overheating of the adipose tissue occurred that often led to fibrous lumps and deep subcutaneous scar tissue. These internal areas of firmness and hardening are now extremely uncommon with sophisticated internal and external thermal monitoring the parameters are adhered to.

12.3 Postinflammatory hyperpigmentation (PIH)

The risk of significant bruising following RFAL assisted liposuction bruising is lessened with RFAL mediated thermal coagulation of small venules and arterioles

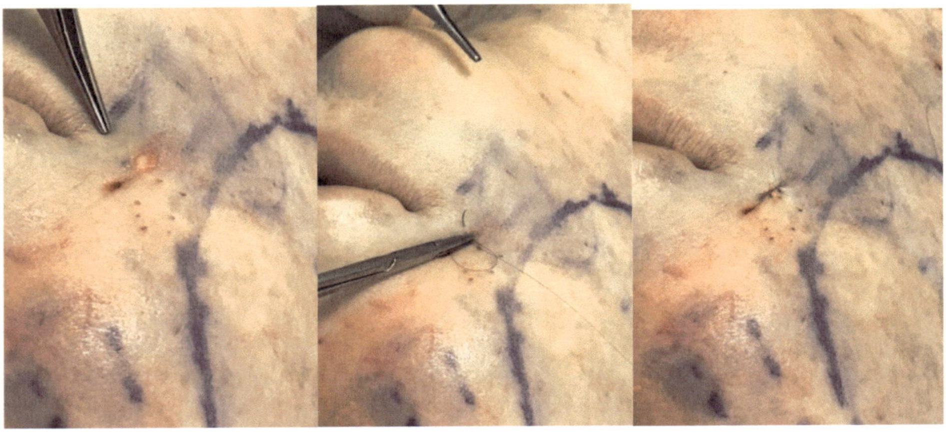

Figure 40.
A small peri-port FaceTite® burn at the entrance of the nasolabial port. Simple epidermal 6–0 nylon closure over the injury will allow subdermal secondary intent healing without an obvious scab. Subsequent fractional RF or laser treatments or, even delayed excision will minimize the risk of any deleterious visible scar.

and the resulting hemosiderin induced PIH is hence far less than lipocontouring with more ecchymosis.

12.4 Seroma

The risk of a seroma is higher using RFAL thermal coagulation is higher, most probably due to a temporary, but reversible injury to the subcutaneous and sub- dermal lymphatic system and so, an internal close drain is used by the author on all abdominal BodyTite® and RFAL cases. BodyTite® and RFAL to other anatomic regions does not increase the risk of seroma, so closed drainage is not deployed.

12.5 Sensory anesthesia

Sensory anesthesia and, to some extent, dysaesthesia is more common with thermal lipocoagulation that non thermal lipoplasty and the during of recovery is longer (more like flap elevation). The reason for the more significant anesthesia is the effect of thermal coagulation resulting in a demyelinating effect of the sensory nerves, but generally 95% of patients get 95% return of sensation.

12.6 Injury to deeper structures

A good working knowledge of the anatomy of the region treated with the BodyTite® applicators will minimize deep internal thermal coagulation of sensitive vascular or neural structures. The most common reported injuries following BodyTite® when looking the worldwide literature would be damage to the antebrachial nerve of the upper arm and typically there's a normal return of sensation, but occasionally permanent anesthesia can occur. Damage to motor nerves should not occur if one performs the RFAL in the correct subcutaneous plane. After 10 years of FaceTite® and AccuTite® to the face and neck, the author does not have a single case of permanent weakness of the marginal mandibular branch of the facial nerve. Because of the thermal containment of the bipolar RFAL, there is little to no heat below the internal electrode, which, when passed above the SMAS, platysma, orbicularis oculi and other facial muscles, the facial nerve is safe. Temporary neuropraxia of the marginal mandibular branch can occur, but this is typically from traction following aspiration and not a thermal injury.

12.7 Prolonged brawny and edema of the skin and dermis

BodyTite® and the RFAL applicators do lead to a more significant soft tissue contraction than any other liposuction assisted device. However, the thermal stimulus stimulation can result in a prolonged thickness and brawny edema of the skin that may take many months to settle. It is been the authors experience that this is uncommon when the focus is deep subcutaneous FSN mediated stimulation, rather than excessive dermal heating. Conservative superficial temperature and end points of 38–40°C are deployed. Because most of the contraction in the body zones relies on the deep FSN and three-dimensional contraction of this FSN, the author generally does not heat closer to the reticular dermis that 1–2 cm. However, when treating in the neck, face and the upper arm, more focus on dermal stimulation is required to gain the contraction and combination with the Morpheus, or RFAL from the "outside in" is safer.

With appropriate patient selection, the risk of excessive skin laxity should be minimal. Most RFAL patients will achieve up to 35% area contraction and reasonable patient selection should result in a significantly high proportion of happy patients that would not have otherwise been liposuction candidates. Perry port burns.

BodyTite® RFAL is a highly sophisticated thermal coagulation system with a multitude of onboard automated, thermally monitored safety systems. It is to a testament to the safety of the system that the tens of thousands of treatments over the past 10 years have resulted in very few serious complications and has made BodyTite® the most effective and safest thermal coagulation body contour tool and in the esthetic space.

13. Conclusions

The BodyTite® workstation has become one of the world's most commonly used thermal coagulation liposuction system. The advantages and opportunities afforded the BodyTite® RFAL physician include:

i. Optimal soft tissue contraction using both the FSN mediated 3D contraction and dermal remodeling.

ii. Studies show upwards of 35% areas contraction after 12 months.

iii. An elegant array of automated feedback thermal control features that minimize over heating of adipose tissue and thermal complications that can ensue.

iv. The ability perform liposuction more effectively on patients with more skin laxity and larger BMI's.

v. The ability to offer outpatient, local anesthesia procedures that combine RFAL and more mini lifts with excellent result, less scarring and downtime.

Conflict of interest

Dr. Mulholland teaches physician workshops on the RFAL technology and is a paid consultant of InMode® and a patent contributor.

Author details

Robert Stephen Mulholland
SpaMedica Plastic Surgery Center (Private Plastic Surgery Practice), Toronto, Canada

*Address all correspondence to: Mulhollandmd@spamedica.com

References

[1] Rohrich RJ, Beran SJ, Kenkel JM, et al. Extending the role of liposuction in body contouring with ultrasound-assisted liposuction. Plastic and Reconstructive Surgery. 1998;**101**: 1090-1102

[2] Zocchi ML. Ultrasonic liposculpturing. Aesthetic Plastic Surgery. 1992;**16**:287-298

[3] Zocchi ML. Ultrasonic assisted lipoplasty: Technical refinements and clinical evaluations. Clinics in Plastic Surgery. 1996;**23**:575-598

[4] DiBernado BE. Randomized, blinded, split abdomen study evaluating skin shrinkage and skin tightening in laser-assisted liposuction versus liposuction control. Aesthetic Surgery Journal. 2010;**30**(4):593-602

[5] Sasaki GH. Quantification of human abdominal tissue tightening and contraction after component treatments with 1064 nm/1320 nm laser-assisted lipolysis: Clinical implications. Aesthetic Surgery Journal. 2010;**30**:239-245

[6] Goldman A. Submental Nd:YAG laser-assisted liposuction. Lasers in Surgery and Medicine. 2006;**38**:181-184

[7] Illouz YG. Body contouring by lipolysis: A 5-year experience with over 3000 cases. Plastic and Reconstructive Surgery. 1983;**72**:591-597

[8] Gasperoni C, Salgarello M, Emiliozzi P, Gargani G. Subdermal liposuction. Aesthetic Plastic Surgery. 1990;**14**: 137-142

[9] Goddio AS. Skin retraction following suction lipectomy by treatment site: A study of 500 procedures in 458 selected subjects. Plastic and Reconstructive Surgery. 1991;**87**:66-75

[10] Matarrasso A. Superficial suction lipectomy: Something old, something new, something borrowed. Annals of Plastic Surgery. 1995;**24**:268-272

[11] Toledo LS. Syringe liposculpturing. Aesthetic Plastic Surgery. 1992;**16**: 287-298

[12] Paul M, Mulholland RS. A new approach for adipose tissue treatment and body contouring using radiofrequency-assisted liposuction. Aesthetic Plastic Surgery (online). 2009. DOI: 10.1007/s00266-009-9342-z

[13] Blugerman G, Schavelzon D, Paul M. A safety and feasibility study of a novel radiofrequency-assisted liposuction technique. Plastic and Reconstructive Surgery. 2010;**125**: 998-1006

[14] Mulholland RS. An in-depth examination of radiofrequency assisted liposuction (RFAL). Journal of Cosmetic Surgery and Medicine. 2009;**4**:14-18

[15] Paul M, Blugerman G, Kreindel M, Mulholland RS. Three-dimensional radiofrequency tissue tightening: A proposed mechanism and applications for body contouring. Aesthetic Plastic Surgery. 2010 (accepted, published with open access)

[16] Duncan DI. Nonexcisional tissue tightening: Creating skin surface area reduction during abdominal liposuction by adding radiofrequency heating. Aesthetic Plastic Surgery. 2013;**33**(8): 1154-1166

[17] Paul MD. Radiofrequency assisted liposuction comes of age: An emerging technology offers an exciting new vista in non-excisional body contouring. Plastic Surgery Practice. 2009;**2**:18-19

[18] Duncan DI. Improving outcomes in upper arm liposuction: Adding radiofrequency-assisted liposuction to

induce skin contraction. Aesthetic Surgery Journal. 2012;**32**(1):84-95

[19] Mulholland RS. Radiofrequency energy for non-invasive and minimally invasive skin tightening. Clinics in Plastic Surgery. 2011;**38**:437-448

[20] Blugerman G, Schalvezon D, Mulholland RS, et al. Gynecomastia treatment using radiofrequency-assisted liposuction (RFAL). European Journal of Plastic Surgery (published online). 2012. DOI: 10.1007/s00238-012-0772-5

[21] Duncan DI. Pilot study using RF assisted tissue tightening for non-excisional breast lifting. In: International Confederation for Plastic, Reconstructive and Aesthetic Surgery, IPRAS. Vol. 9, Issue 8. 2012. p. 76

[22] Divaris M, Boisnic S, Branchet MC, Paul MD. A clinical and histological study of radiofrequency-assisted liposuction (RFAL) mediated skin tightening and cellulite improvement. Journal of Cosmetics, Dermatological Sciences and Applications. 2011;**1**:36-42

Chapter 5

Vaser Body Contouring Achieving a More Defined Shape

Alberto Di Giuseppe, Federico Giovagnoli, Saverio Di Giuseppe and Diana Ronconi

Abstract

The art of body shaping has changed in the last decade, with the new philosophy of superficial sculpturing and fat removal and fat adding in combination. Vaser ultrasound device allows a superficial undermining of the skin all over the body; deeper fat removal allows precise contouring. Fat harvesting with new device allows harvesting and concentrating high-quality fat, which is added in zones to enhance curvature and balance of body shape.

Keywords: vaser liposuction, fat harvesting, fat transfer, superficial sculpturing

1. Introduction

The evolution of body shaping techniques in the last decades has affected new technologies as well as vaser ultrasound liposuction; new blunt and narrow cannulas, which replaced sharp, larger diameter ones; and wet and superwet infiltrations which have replaced aggressive dry liposuction. Moreover, the art of fat harvesting and fat transfer, combined with the new studies of stem cell and their capability of generating new tissues, has led to a more sophisticated way to intend the art of body contouring. The new vision has a more artistic impact on the tridimensional sculpture of body frame. Another fundamental issue has been the understanding of the skin retraction capabilities enhanced by new technologies and the importance of full understanding of the anatomy of body muscles to help define and shape the body.

2. Heading section

New technologies have entered the market in the last decade, as power-assisted technology, ultrasound technology, and laser technology, in order to facilitate fat removal, reduce trauma, and improve skin retraction. I have personally been one of the pioneers of ultrasound-assisted liposuction since they appeared in the early 2000s and contributed to the realization of the new vaser device, more advanced and safer than previous ultrasound-assisted devices in commerce 20 years ago. In vaser technology (**Figure 1**), vaser is an acronym of vibration amplification sound at resonance and is a third generation of ultrasound-assisted liposuction that uses ultrasound energy to melt fat tissue, ultrasound technology emulsifies the fat for removal in such a delicate way that preserves as much of the tissue of the matrix as possible while emulsifying the desired amount of fatty tissue. Special titanium probes deliver the ultrasound energy to fat tissue, after proper infiltration with tumescent solution, allowing the selective destruction of only the fat tissue through three mechanisms: (1) cavitation, (2) mechanical, and (3) thermal.

In cavitation effect (**Figure 2**), the vaser probes vibrate at ultrasonic frequencies creating compressive and rarefactive forces around the grooved tip; cavitation microbubbles expand and then implode, releasing energy that disrupts the adipocyte architecture until an emulsion of fat and fluid is formed.

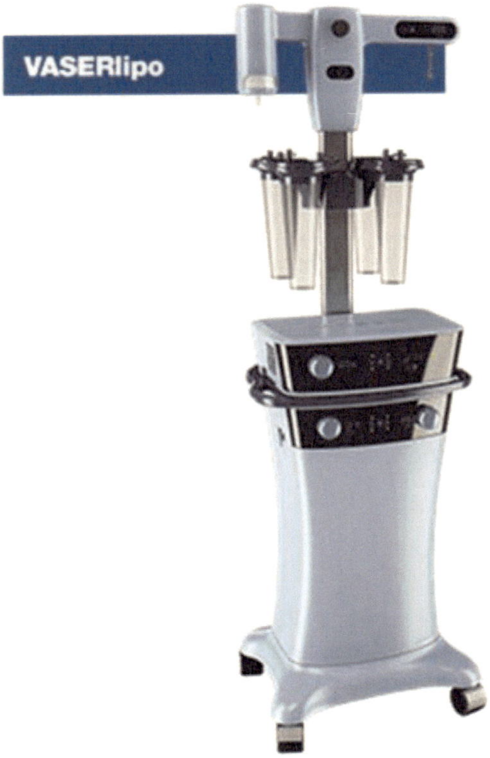

Figure 1.
Vaser system.

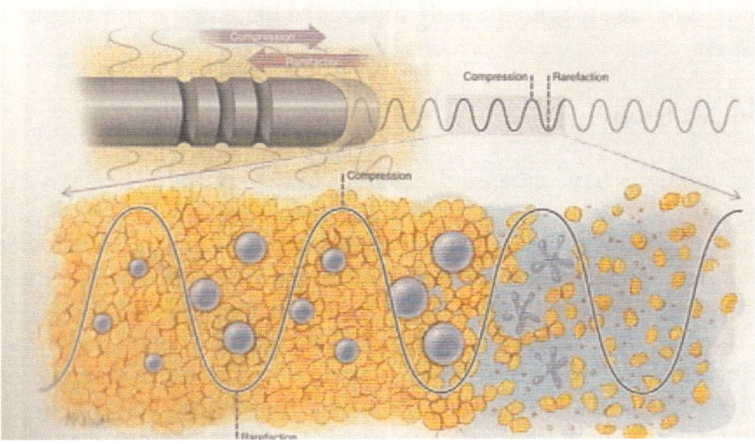

Figure 2.
Cavitation.

Mechanical disruption of fat occurs at the tip of the probe, where the vibrating metal surface comes in contact with the adipocytes. Cavitation and mechanical disruption of adipose tissue occur due to relative fragility of this tissue compared to other tissues such as vessels, muscle, and nerves. This is why this process is safe and effective, spears the connective and vascular network of the skin and subcutaneous tissue, allows a safe subcutaneous superficial undermining of the skin, and is thus a major skin retraction of tissue. The thinnest is the dermal tissue, the highest is the skin retraction, and liposuction is the term to define vaser smoothening of the fat. Careful emulsification, not an aggressive fat removal, is selective where needed in two different layers: subcutaneous for superficial definition and deep dermal for volume removal.

Minding the advantages of this technology, the plastic surgeon must be able to achieve superior results in terms of definition and shaping.

1. With superficial fattening and careful undermining, he can achieve a thin layer of skin flap, ideal for superior skin retraction.

2. Deeper fat removal can be done in a less traumatic mode, leaving less scar tissue, with less chances of seroma formation and induration and asymmetry.

3. Fat removal can be accomplished with fat preservation, harvesting, and preparation for further implant. Fat emulsified still contains the same amount of viable adipocytes as in standard liposuction, with same stem-derived cells that are vital to enhance fat survival rate when transferred to target areas (breast, thighs, buttocks, face, etc.).

All those potential weapons must be utilized by surgeon to better define the body shape and achieve better contouring [1, 2].

3. Fat anatomy

The subcutaneous tissue is divided into three layers: a superficial adipose tissue layer, an intermediate membranous layer, and a deep adipose tissue.

The thickness and proportion of those layers vary throughout the body depending on the anatomic region: the abdominal has a prominent fascial plane, making it easier to distinguish between the two fatty layers.

In the leg, there is an attenuated fibrous membrane which separates from the muscle fascia. In the trunk, the adipose tissue is similar, as in gross appearance and density and structure (**Figure 3**).

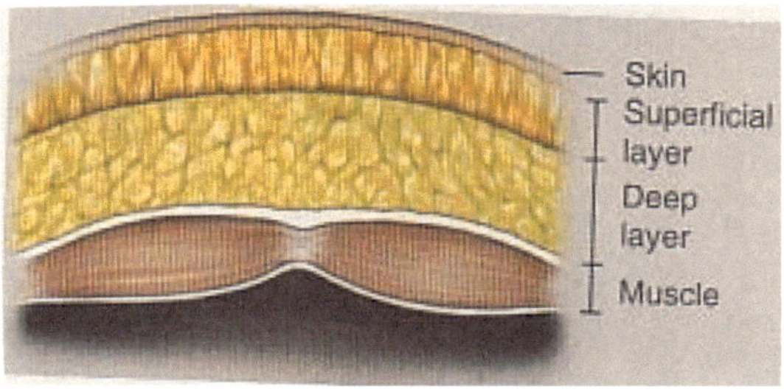

Figure 3.
Fat anatomy.

In the thighs and gluteus, the subcutaneous fascia fuses with the gluteal crease and intergluteal fold [3].

4. Surgeon ability in shaping

The introduction of vaser allows efficient and safe emulsification of fat in superficial and deep layers while preserving vascular and neural structures.

This is a new chisel in surgeon hands to sculpture the body as a work of the artist, working in all subcutaneous planes, by adding and subtracting fat with delicate instruments and refined techniques. The subdermal plane is no longer a taboo area; controlled deformities are desirable, and muscular definition is attainable through lipoplasty by revealing the underlying anatomy.

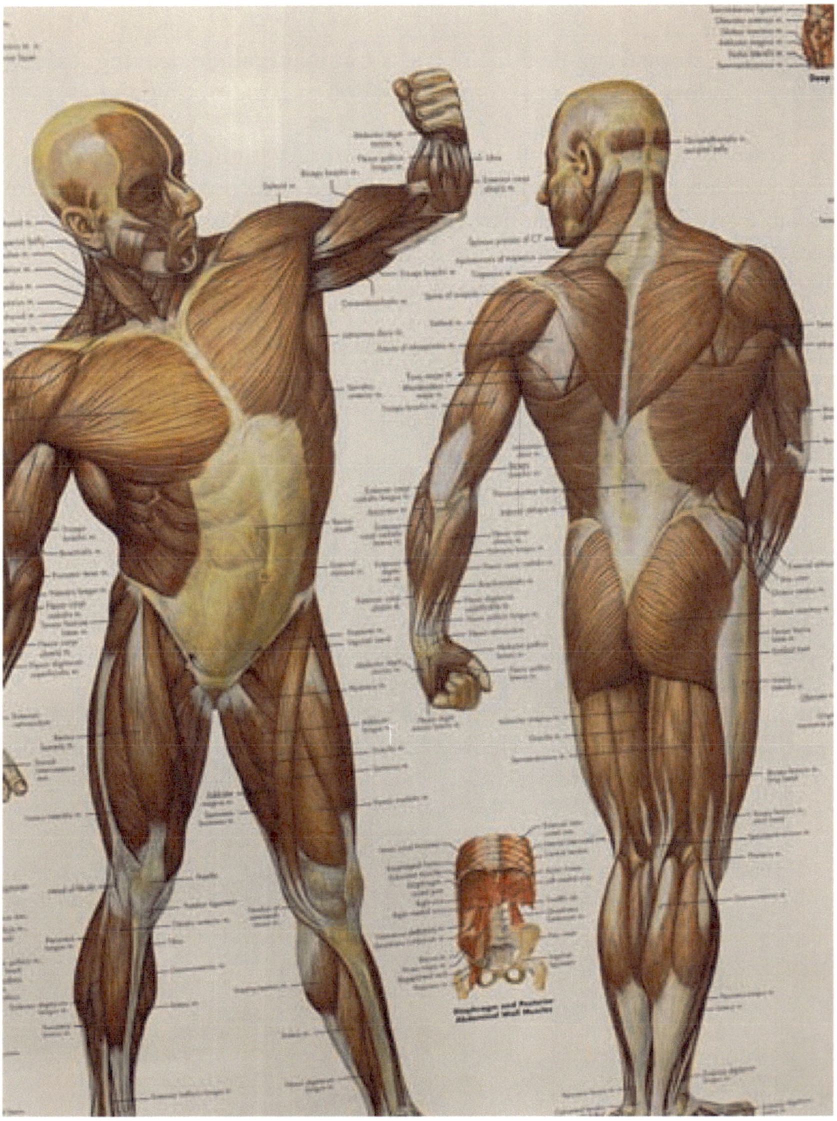

Figure 4.
Muscle anatomy.

The full understanding of muscle anatomy is essential to try to recreate a muscle-shaped body and enhance definition and contouring (**Figure 4**).

The lines of body are described as natural curves which are defined by muscle, bone frame, and fat deposit. Posture is another component to assess the natural body appearance, and man and woman are different of course. Lipoplasty can address only subcutaneous tissue and is not a solution for abdominal protrusion secondary to muscle weakness or intraabdominal fat. This will require muscle exercise and diet to compensate. The achievement of symmetry and proportion is the goal of any body contouring procedure. The man of Vitruvio, designed by Leonardo da Vinci, remains the golden reference of human proportions. In the recent age, new trends in fashion have defined new more athletic figure, more toned, even in woman, answering to the so popular attended gym all over the world.

The surgeon view and sense of artistry are essential in planning a good shaped body. He must create in his mind a tridimensional view of the new body to shape: ideally must thin the subcutaneous tissues as much as to display and reveal the superficial musculature, removing fat and highlighting major muscle groups. The salient features of the muscular anatomy relevant to body contouring are outlined such as origin, insertion, orientation, form created, and relationship to adjacent muscle groups.

Main muscles involved are the rectus muscles, the oblique muscle, the pectoralis in the front appearance, the latissimus dorsi, the lumbaris, and the gluteus in the back.

The muscle edges and the intermuscular digitations must be outlined to better define an athletic abdomen, together with the linea alba and linea semilunaris recreation.

Lines of transition between muscles must be obtained with more suction in a superficial manner. The main concept is removing and revealing what is underneath in normal-weighted patient, while traditional liposuction focuses in removing fat in overweight patient. The sculpturing surgeon tries to reveal the underlying musculature and body anatomy; shaping is a combination of removal to reveal what is underneath and adding in areas of deficiency to give more curvature.

It is a mixture of light and shadow and depression and concavities to give the impression of more defined and toned body. In man, fullness is desirable in the upper pectoral region, deltoid, and biceps, and frequently, fat is grafted to augment the pectoralis and deltoids. In woman, the buttocks and breasts often require augmentation to improve fullness and increase curves.

An example of this high-definition surgery in man is given:

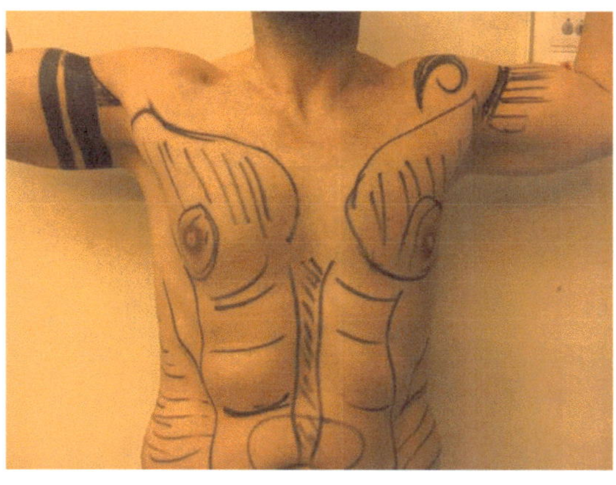

Figure 5.
Planning high-definition frontal view.

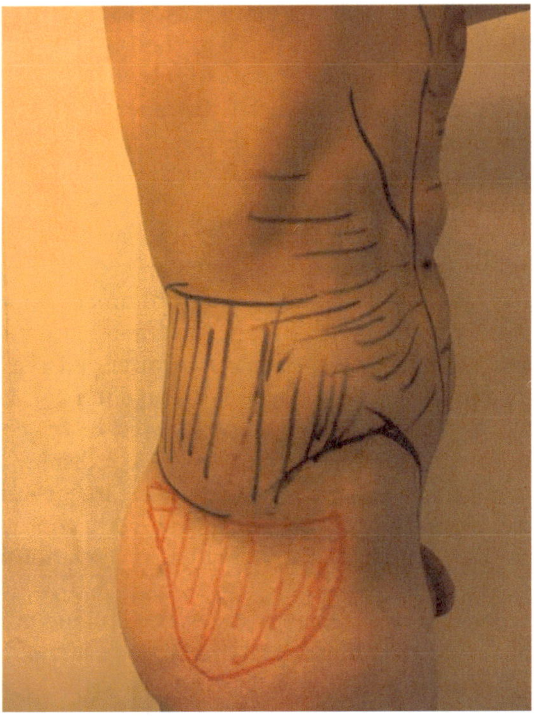

Figure 6.
Planning of lateral side. Margin of the oblique muscle outlined, edge of latissimus muscle, the inguinal ligament, and in red the outer medium gluteus zone to be grafted with fat to increase roundness.

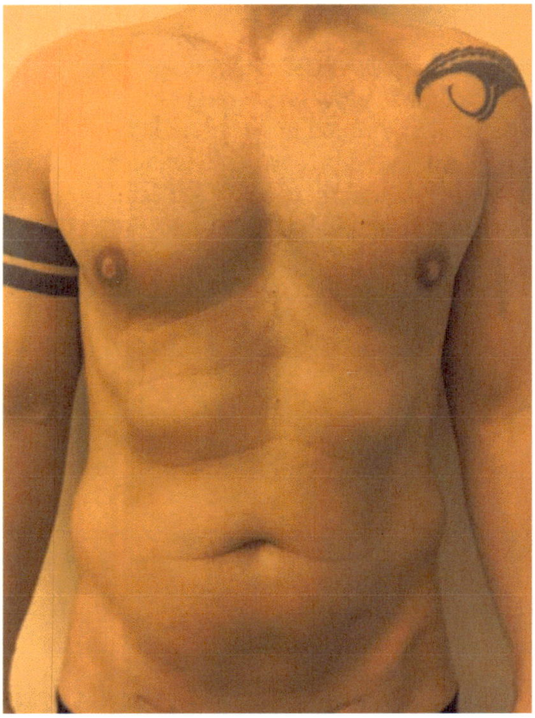

Figure 7.
Preop appearance.

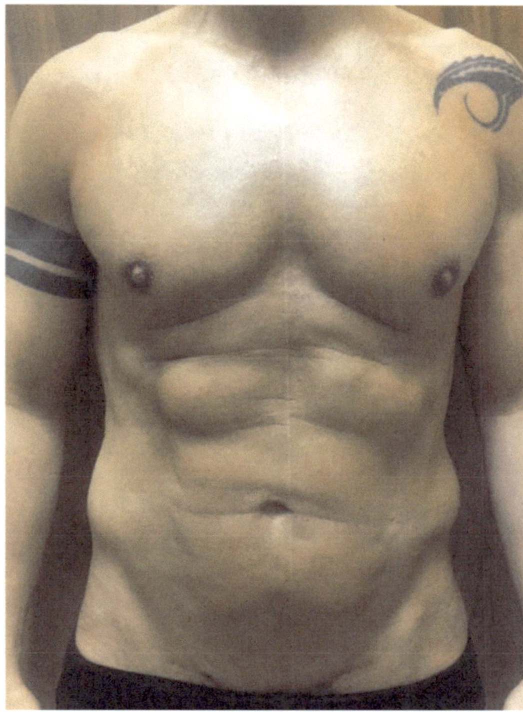

Figure 8.
Postop appearance at 3 months.

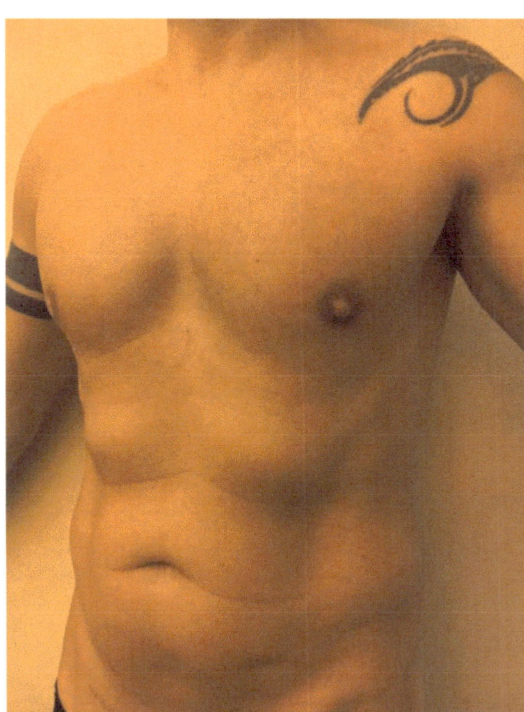

Figure 9.
Preop oblique view.

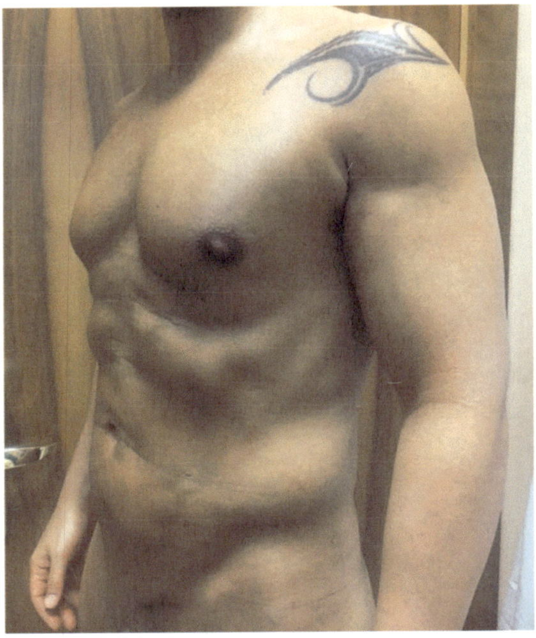

Figure 10.
Postop oblique view.

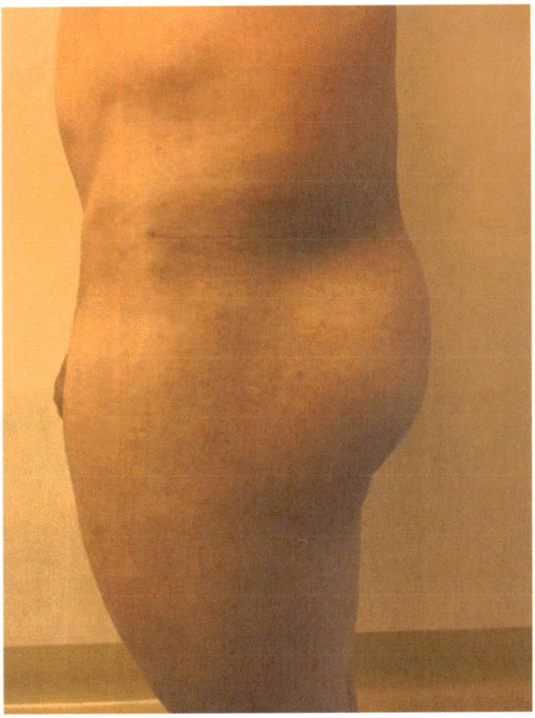

Figure 11.
Pregluteal definition and torso contouring.

32-year-old athletic body, looking for definition (**Figure 5**).

The areas of biceps muscle are marked, the area of male gland reduction is circled, the area of superficial fattening of male breast is marked, and the area of fat transfer to pectoralis muscle to add volume is marked as well.

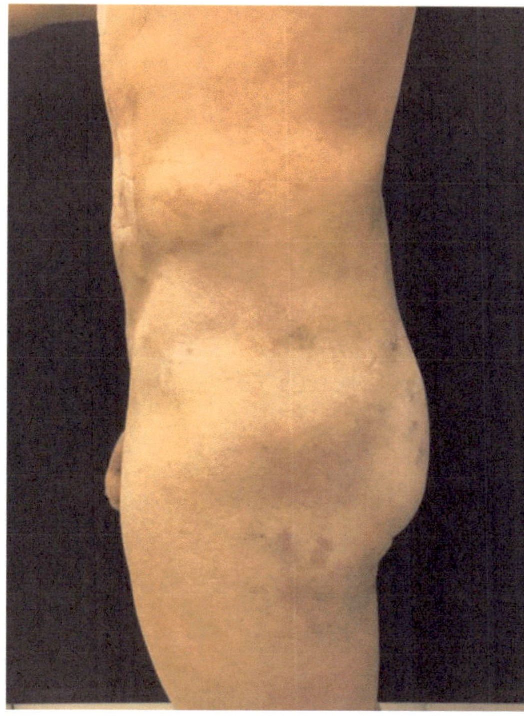

Figure 12.
Postgluteal definition and torso contouring.

The linea alba is marked in the central abdomen; the outer margin of the rectus muscle and the interdigitations of the muscle area are marked as well.

The margin of the oblique muscles, the inguinal ligament to create a marked depression, and the extra fat surrounding the navel are circled, and finally, the lateral flanks are lined where fat needs to be removed (**Figure 6**) [3, 4].

Result of definition of an athletic young body is shown, after linea alba and linea semilunaris deepening and oblique muscle and inguinal ligament being enhanced.

Note the concavities and shadows created with false deformities to give more power and more density to muscle areas (**Figures 7–10**).

The gluteal region is approached in a distinct way: lateral flanks are reduced in an aggressive way; the inguinal ligament is enhanced and glutes' prominence reduced, while the outer medium gluteus muscle is filled to improve athletic definition (**Figures 11** and **12**).

5. Woman contouring

Woman body is different from man body, in human form, bone shape, muscle density, and fat distribution. Hormones influence woman body through all life and are responsible for fat distribution changes and shape changes.

Maternity affects body volume and shape as well, with radical changes which need to be addressed in body contouring surgery.

Forty-five-year-old lady had two pregnancies and never regained young body appearance after first pregnancy from preop figure, flanks appear large, abdomen is fatty, and there are no lines, no curvature, and no definition in body shape.

The posterior trunk appears heavy, and back rolls are located in the middle of the trunk.

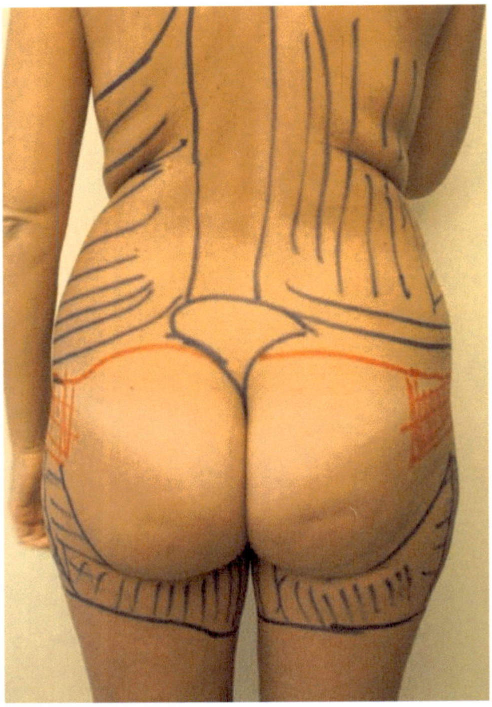

Figure 13.
Planning.

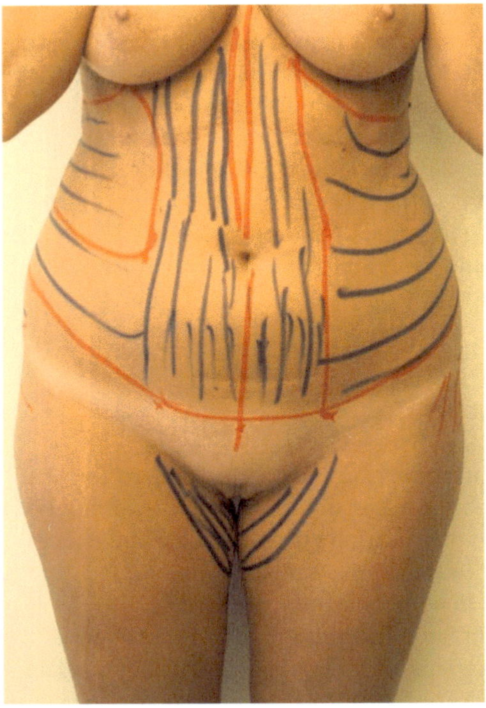

Figure 14.
Planning.

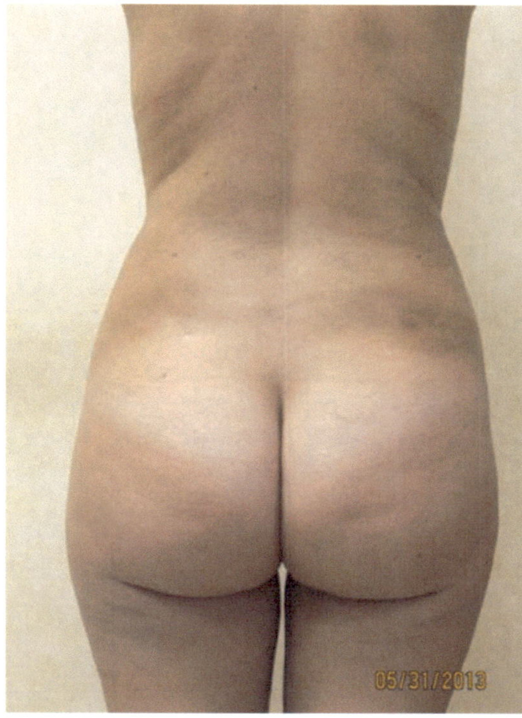

Figure 15.
Preop.

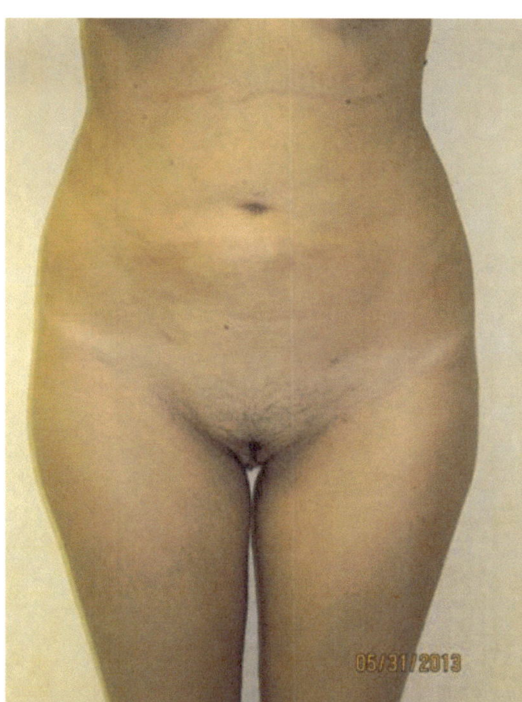

Figure 16.
Postop.

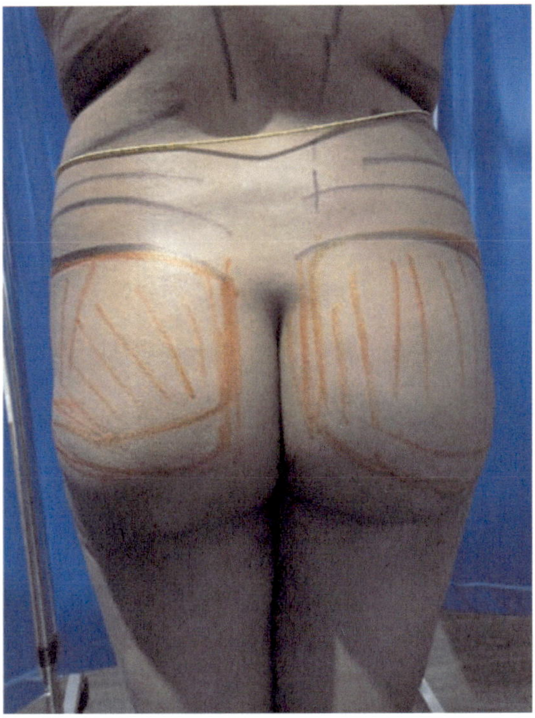

Figure 17.
Planning of fat removal.

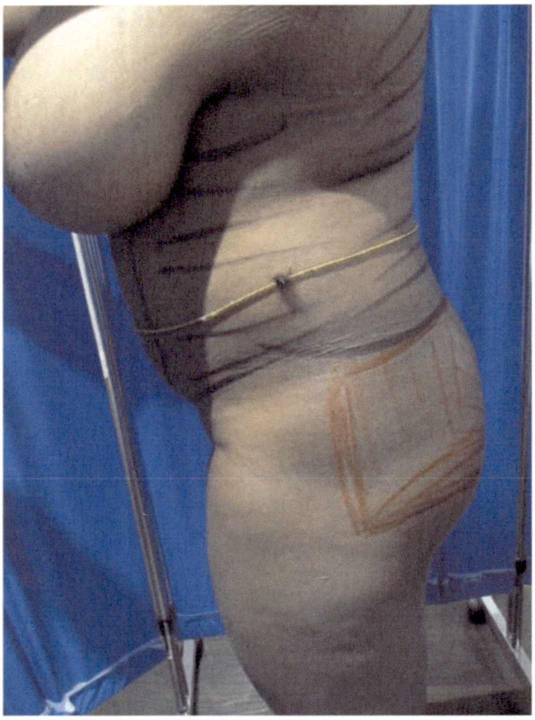

Figure 18.
Planning of buttocks fat grafting.

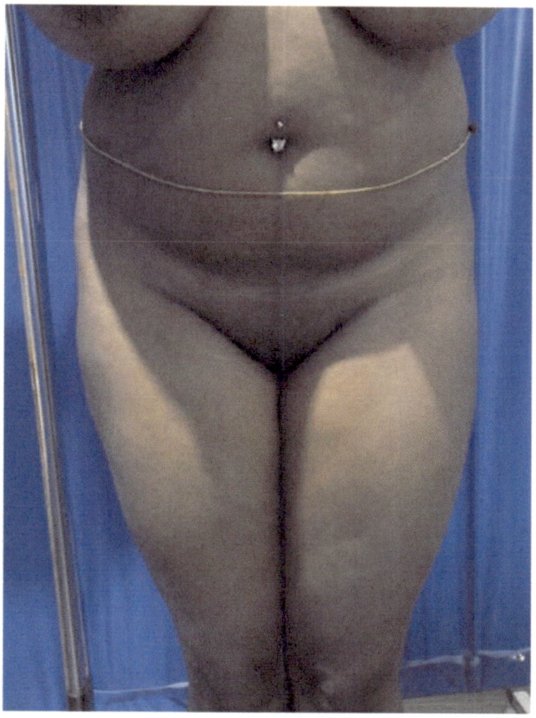

Figure 19.
Preop.

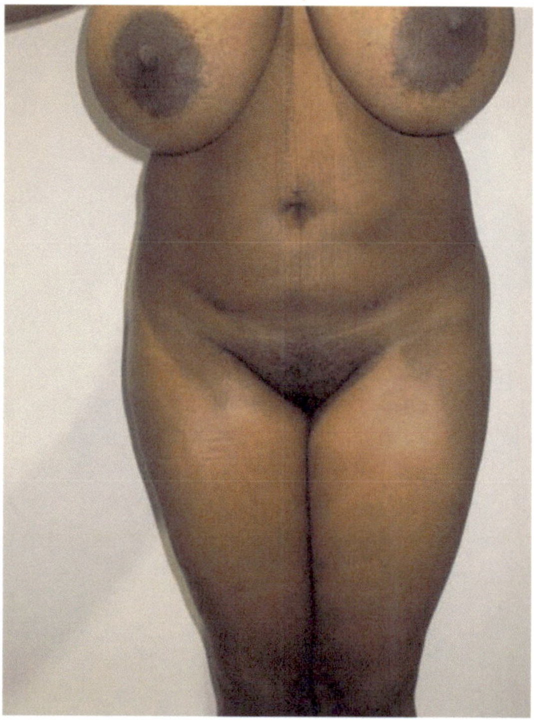

Figure 20.
Postop 3 months.

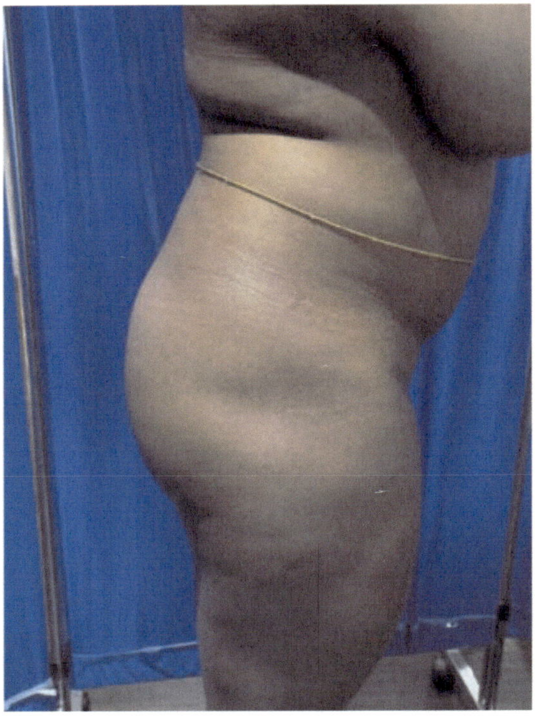

Figure 21.
Pre- and immediate postop result after 1400 ml fat grafting buttocks.

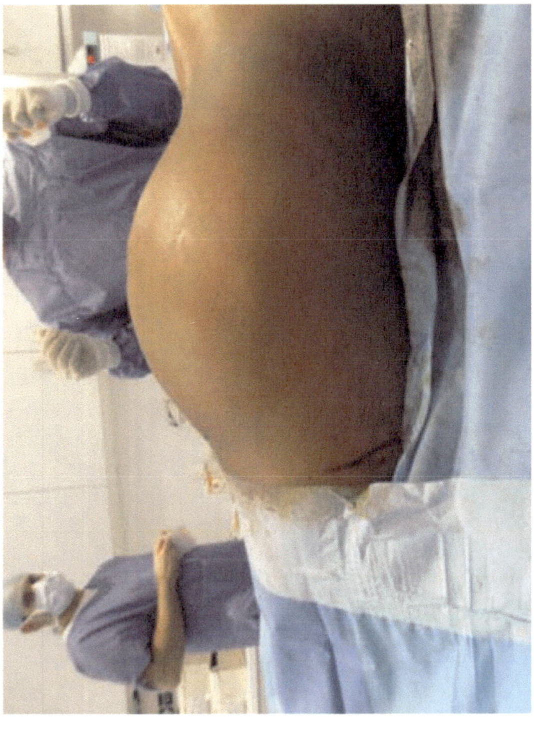

Figure 22.
Pre- and immediate postop result after 1400 ml fat grafting buttocks.

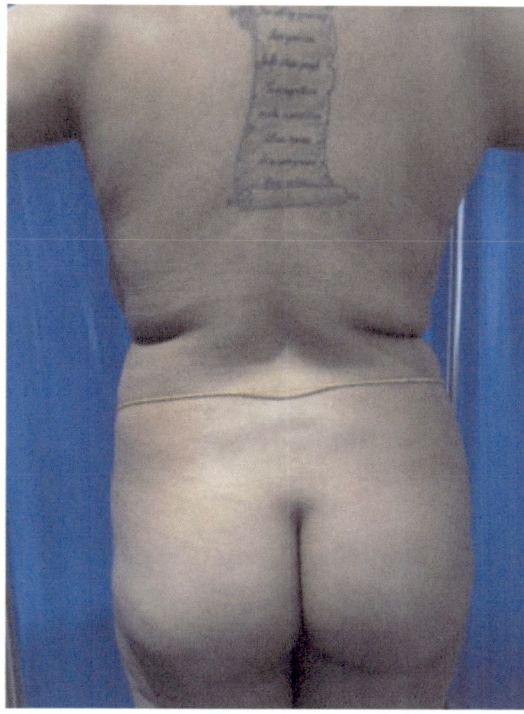

Figure 23.
Pre- and immediate postop result after 1400 ml fat grafting buttocks.

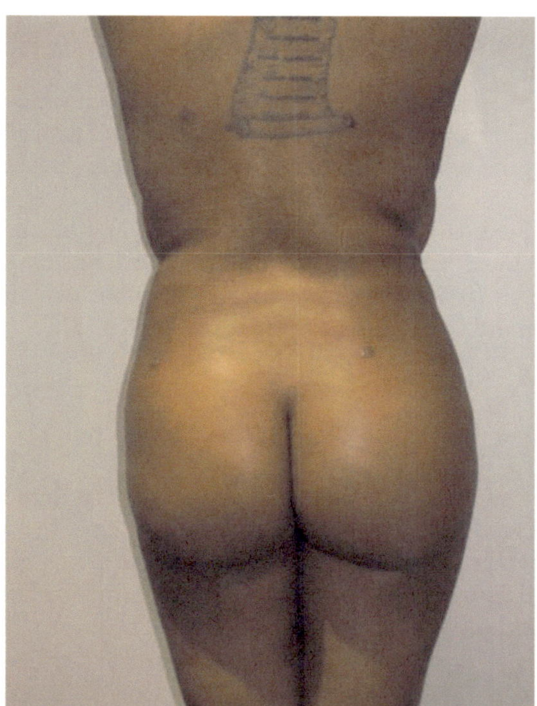

Figure 24.
Pre- and immediate postop result after 1400 ml fat grafting buttocks.

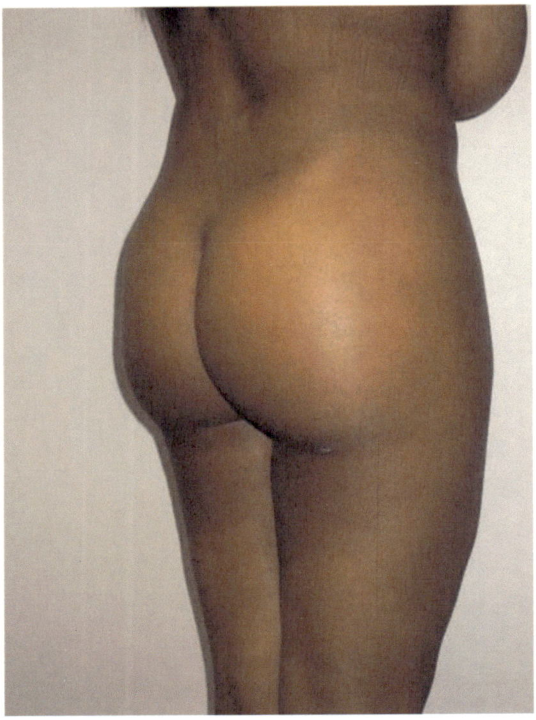

Figure 25.
Pre- and immediate postop result after 1400 ml fat grafting buttocks.

Vaser liposuction is planned, with definition of anterior rectus muscle, flattening, and contouring and reshaping back and creating more female lines (**Figures 13–16**).

About 4000 ml of fat is removed from anterior upper and lower abdomen, back and flanks, and inner thighs.

Buttocks area is one of the most requested by women nowadays. Reshaping means enhancing volume and giving more roundness and projection. Women are often lucky to have enough donor fat areas from abdomen, posterior trunk, and flanks.

This 28-year-old woman asked for body reshaping and buttock enhancement.

Vaser liposuction was performed, 4500 ml removed, and 1500 ml of fat harvested and then grafted to buttocks, outer and top buttock areas.

Results after 3 months are presented (**Figures 17–25**) [5].

6. Conclusion

Body contouring surgery has changed deeply in the last decade—new technologies, more sophisticated technique—and has led to superior result in terms of definition. This is an art and must be considered in this way—plastic surgeon is a sculpturing boy and uses his chisel and talent to shape in a tridimensional space using fat removal and fat enhancement.

Conflict of interest

The authors have no conflicts of interest to declare.

Author details

Alberto Di Giuseppe[1,2,3*], Federico Giovagnoli[4], Saverio Di Giuseppe[5] and Diana Ronconi[5]

1 Department of Plastic Surgery, University of Padova, Italy

2 Private Practice, London, UK

3 Private Practice, Bologna, Italy

4 Liceo Galilei Ancona, Italy

5 Faculty of Medicine and Surgery, University of Rome, Italy

*Address all correspondence to: albertodigiuseppemd@gmail.com

References

[1] Shiffman MA, Di Giuseppe A, editors. Body Contouring. DOI: 10.1007/978-3-642-02639-3

[2] Rubin JP, Jewell ML, Richter DF, Uebel CO, editors. Body Contouring and Liposuction. DOI: 10.1007/978-1-4557-3796-3

[3] Shiffman MA, Di Giuseppe A, Bassetto F, editors. Stem Cells in Aesthetic Procedures. DOI: 10.1007/978-3-642-45207-9

[4] Shiffman MA, Di Giuseppe A, editors. Liposuction. 2nd ed. DOI: 10.1007/978-3-662-48903-1

[5] Hoyos AE, Prendergast PM, editors. High Definition Body Sculpting. DOI: 10.1007/978-3-642-54891-8

Chapter 6

Creating the Ideal Buttock (Lifting, Implanting or Fat Grafting)

Angelo Cuzalina and Armando Retana

Abstract

An attractive buttock has become more popular than ever before owing to social media and popular iconic celebrity figures. For many women today, a full, well-rounded buttock is considered attractive and has connotations of health, youthfulness, as well as sexual allure. There are a host of choices that can be used to improve buttock shape, tightness and size including non-surgical injections, implants, fat, skin removal, liposuction and various energy devices. Understanding the diagnosis is critical to formulate an ideal plan and then select the best technique. This chapter will cover the top three surgical procedures in great detail; the formal buttock lift, the Brazilian butt lift (BBL) and gluteal implants.

Keywords: Brazilian butt lift, buttock augmentation, gluteoplasty, butt implant, fat grafting

1. Introduction

An attractive buttock has become extremely popular in the last decade thanks to social media and some popular iconic figures that make a living simply from have what many thinks of as a "nice butt." However, before the recent surg in popularity, various gluteal shaping procedure have been performed over the past half century to correct deformities and improve patient' proportions, laxity or size. Most of the procedures remain about the same but many patient's idea of what a beautiful backside should look like has changed. Still, physiologically, the buttock remains a major weight bearing anatomic unit as well as a source for moment and strength. It has been the source of inspiration by many artists. Yet, many cultures use the buttocks as the site for corporal punishment. In numerous cultures the buttock plays a significant role in sexual attraction and seduction. A full, well-rounded buttocks is considered attractive because it indicates health, youthfulness, and could indirectly be related to fertility, as a larger pelvic is considered more ideal for childbearing.

There are a multitude of options that can be used to improve the buttock including non-surgical injections, implants, fat, excisional, liposuction and various energy devices (**Figure 1**). Understand the diagnosis helps formulate the ideal plan and selection of the best technique to give the patient a pleasing result. This chapter will cover the top three surgical procedures in great detail; the formal buttock lift, the Brazilian butt lift (BBL) and gluteal implants (**Figure 2**). Currently, more than ever, the buttock plays a significant role in physical and sexual attraction. This particular body part has gained an enormous amount of attention in social media

IntechOpen

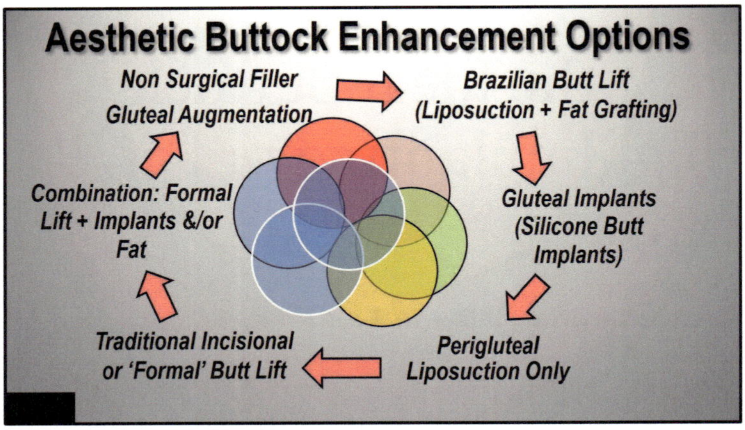

Figure 1.
Enhancing the buttock can be performed via a wide variety of options. Understanding the diagnosis is critical to select the proper technique for buttock enhancement.

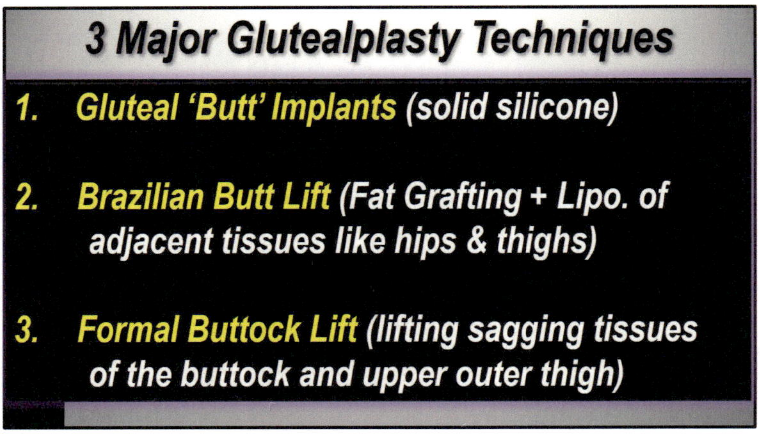

Figure 2.
Not including filler injections, the top three surgical gluteal enhancement or 'gluteoplasty' procedures are Brazilian butt lifting (BBL), formal or skin excisional buttock lifting as well gluteal implant placement.

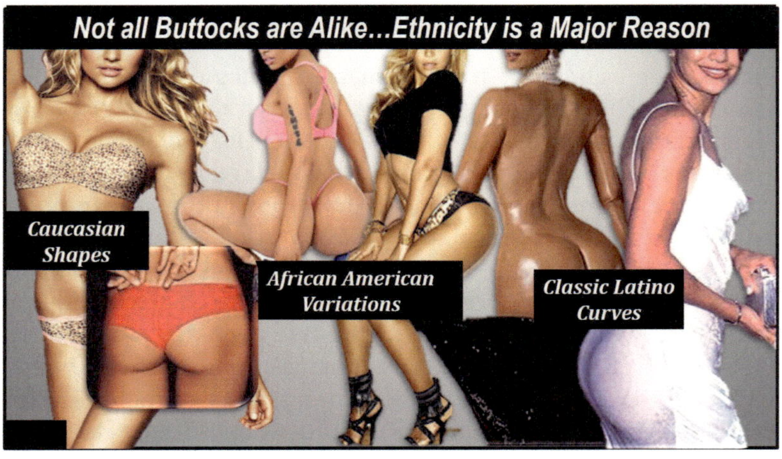

Figure 3.
The buttock has gained a lot of attention in social media and conventional media due to a number of Hollywood celebrities and the rising popularity of social media models who flaunt their extreme curves in the gluteal area in particular. This has caused an exponential rise in buttock cosmetic surgery procedures in the last decade.

and conventional media due to a number of Hollywood celebrities and the rising popularity of social media models in recent years causing a spike in gluteal enhancement operations (**Figure 3**).

2. Universal proportions and characteristics of a beautiful buttocks

When it comes to body contouring surgery, the surgeon should know the universal characteristics and proportions that make up a universally attractive buttock.

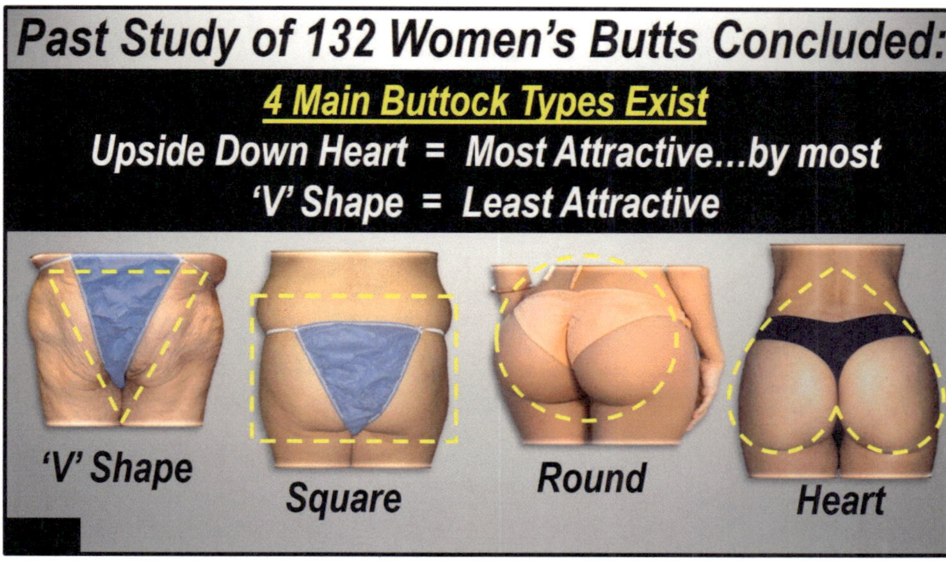

Figure 4.
The most common four buttock shapes are considered to be the round, square, 'V' shape, and the upside-down heart With the upside down heart in general being most attractive and the V shape, also known as a frog's buttock' as being least attractive as well as the hardest to correct.

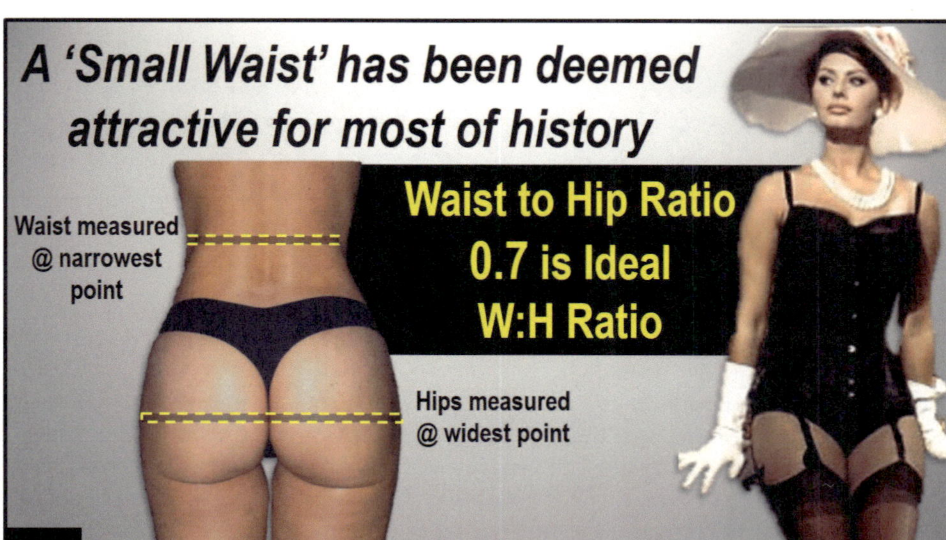

Figure 5.
Throughout history, a small waist has generally been considered attractive. A specific waist-to-hip ratio of 0.7 appears most attractive.

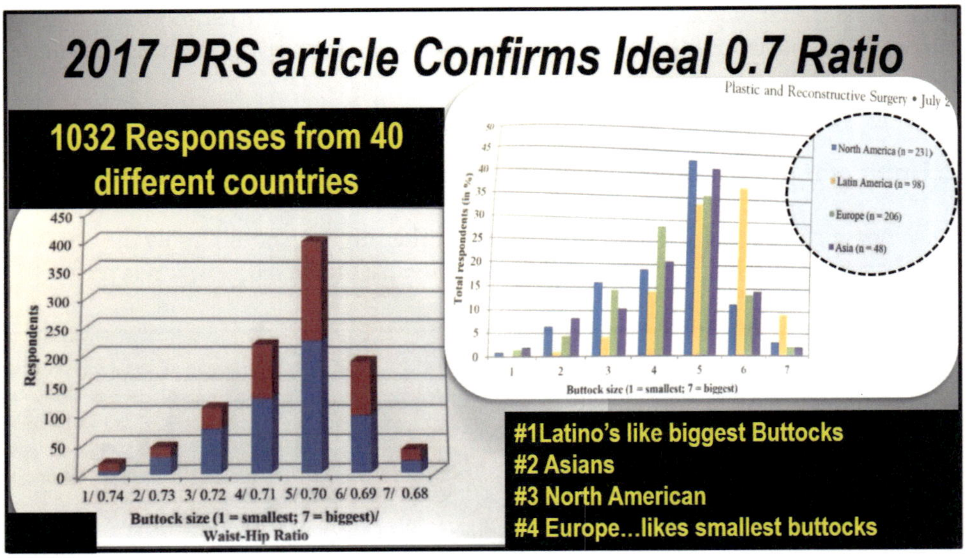

Figure 6.
Several studies recently validated that the ideal female figure has a waist-to-hip ratio of 0.7, yet they also found ethnic differences in what size buttock various cultures found attractive.

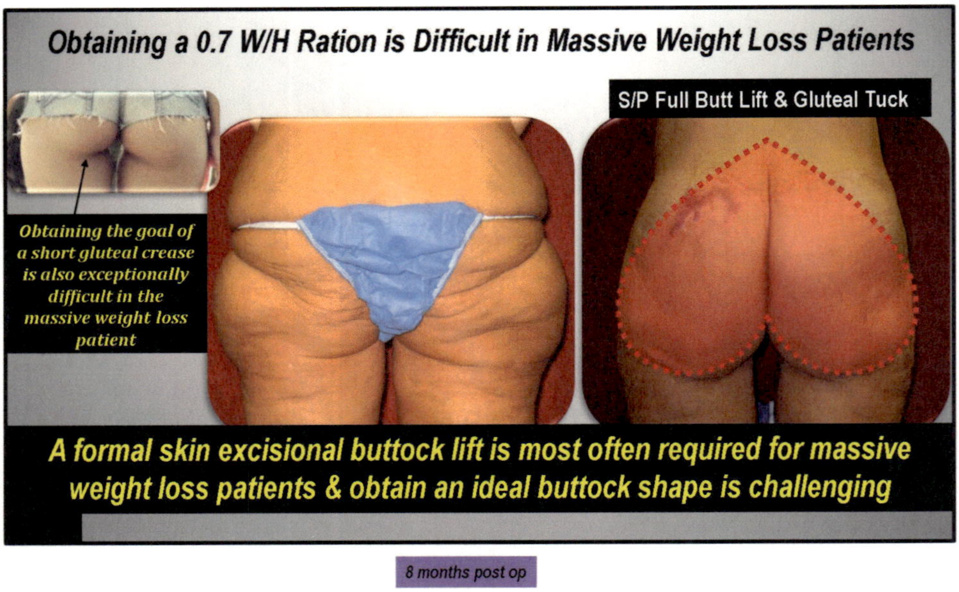

Figure 7.
Massive weight loss patients often require formal skin excision buttock lifts plus augmentation. Even with maximum effort, it is difficult to achieve a small waist, short infra gluteal crease and upside-down heart shape.

Many have classified buttock into shape categories. The most common four are the round, square, "V" shape, and the upside-down heart (**Figure 4**). With the upside-down heart in general being most attractive and the V shape being least attractive. In 1993, Singh published his study on the role that the waist-to-hip ratio plays in regards to female physical attractiveness in the Journal of Personality and Social Psychology [1]. After the analysis of three different studies, Singh proposed that there is a correlation between female attractiveness and the proportions of the waist and buttocks which he described as the waist-to-hip ratio (WHR). Moreover, he found that males in those studies considered female figures with a low WHR more attractive, healthier, and of greater reproductive potential than females with higher WHR. More specifically, the studies indicated that the ideal female figure has a waist-to-hip ratio of 0.7 (**Figure 5**). This ratio is measured by obtaining the circumference of the waist at its narrowest area and dividing it by the circumference of the thighs ("hips") at the level of the buttocks with maximum projection (**Figure 6**). Another characteristic of a beautiful, youthful, and attractive buttocks includes a short gluteal crease that does not extend past the medial third with no ptosis over this line. Such idea buttock shapes may be a goal for many but can be exceptional hard to achieve in some patients such as massive weight loss clientele (**Figure 7**).

3. Ethnic variations for an attractive buttock

It is fair to say that all cultures find a female body with a waist-to-hip ratio around 0.7 to be very attractive. However, there are significant ethnic differences when it comes to the ideal shape of a buttock. The senior author has performed well over 1000 gluteal augmentations including fat grafting, gluteal lifts and gluteal implants. It is our experience that patient's satisfaction depends heavily on what their ethnicity perceives as an attractively shaped buttock and did the surgeons results match what they hoped to achieve. If the surgeon does not understand how significant the buttock shape is based on ethnicity, a good result from the surgeon's standpoint may be a terrible result for the patient. This observation is based on over 22 years' experience performing gluteal surgeries in many parts of the world and on an extremely large number of ethnically diverse patients (**Figure 8**). With the United States and the world as a whole becoming much more diverse due to immigration patterns and medical tourism, it is important for the surgeon to take into consideration ethnic background of the patient when doing this type of surgery. It is also important to go over before and after photos with patients to assess what it is that they consider ideal for their body. The major differences noted among ethnic groups are:

1. **Caucasian female** patients prefer an average fullness but not extremely large in most cases as a general rule of thumb. They like their fullness in the upper

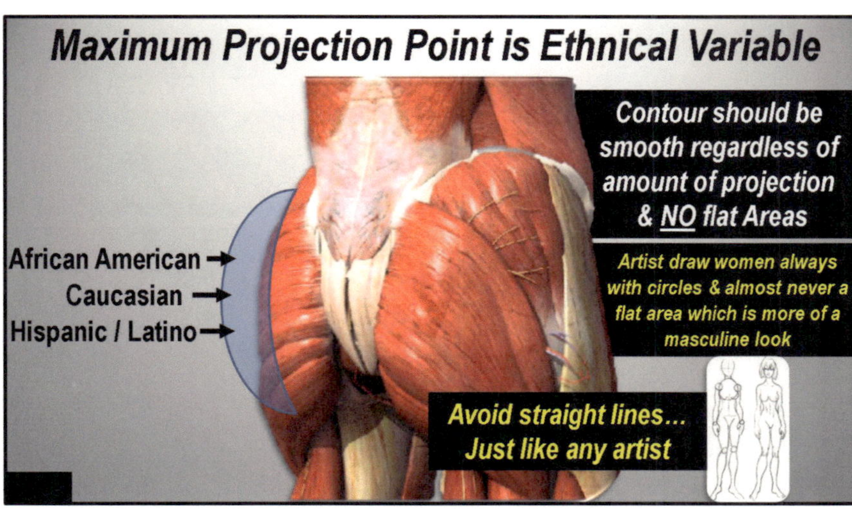

Figure 8.
Ethnic diversity regarding buttock shape is particularly significant for differences seen between Caucasian, Latinos, and African American women. Maximum projection location is one difference among this group as shown and lateral fullness is another area where Caucasian vary greatly from Latinos or Black women.

to middle third of the buttocks and like an overall upside-down heart shape. However, most Caucasian patients do not like the fullness in the lateral thigh and if it is present, they often request liposuction of this area the call the lateral thigh fat immediately below the greater trochanter depression, "saddlebags". This same area may be referred to as "hips" by a Latino or Black patient which may be confusing if not understood. Typically, Caucasians like a slimmer and more athletic look to their buttocks (**Figure 9**).

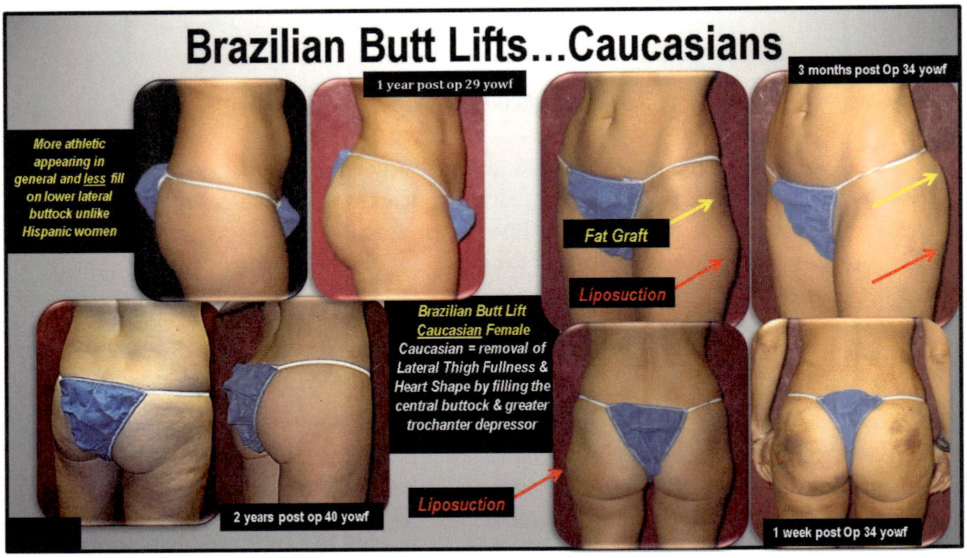

Figure 9.
BBLs for Caucasian women often require removing a portion of the convexity as shown in the lateral thigh fat not typically removed in Latinos or Blacks. Fat can be grafting into the lateral greater trochanter depression but more grafting in general is focused centrally versus laterally.

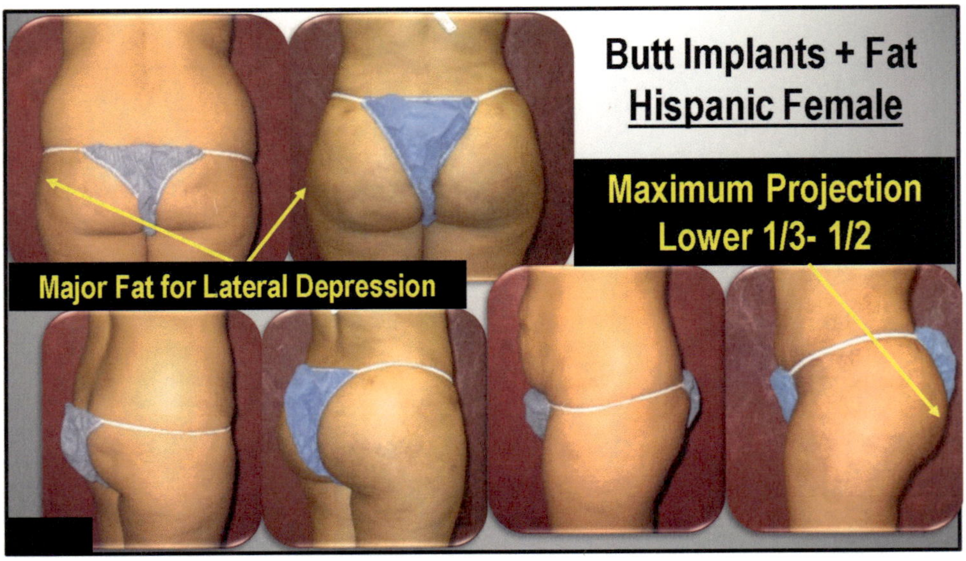

Figure 10.
BBLs for Latino / Hispanic women typically involves significant fat grafting to the mid and lower 1/3 of the buttock as well as major grafting in the lower lateral buttock. Even when a large implant is used, many Hispanic women will also want additional fill laterally with fat to accentuate the upside-down heart shape.

2. Patients of **Hispanic or South American** decent prefer a buttock that is very full (larger volumes than most Caucasians) with significant additional fullness in the lateral buttocks and also in the lateral thigh area (**Figure 10**). For the most part, they prefer their maximum point of projection in the lower one half to one third of the buttocks. The preferred shape among this ethnic group is an extreme upside-down heart with more fullness in the lateral thigh area. Unlike Caucasian patients, liposuction of the lateral thigh area is almost never desired in Black or Hispanic women (**Figure 11**).

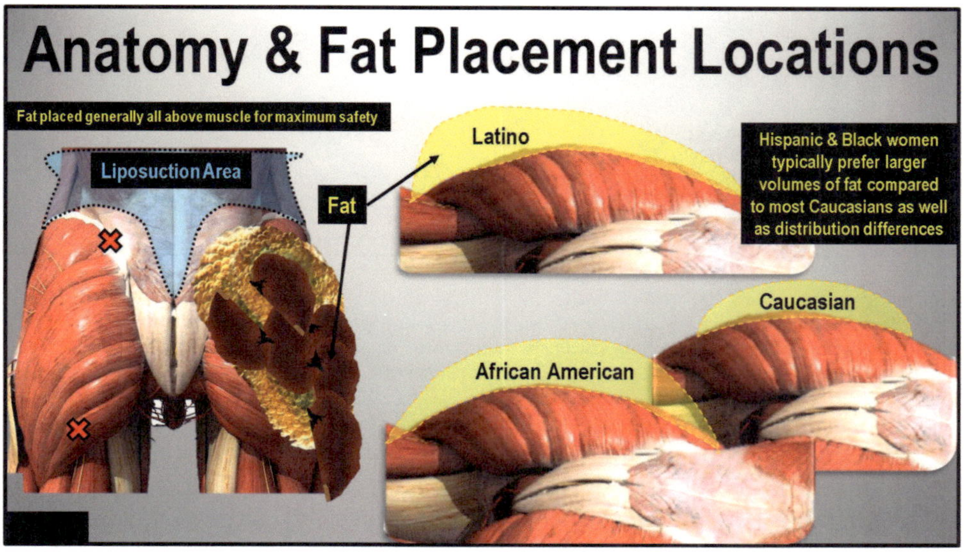

Figure 11.
This figure demonstrate the fat grafting pattern commonly seen with differing ethnicities from a more lateral view. Black and Hispanic females generally prefer larger volumes than Caucasian women but Black women like more rounded appearance with a more accentuated Lordotic curve from back to buttock.

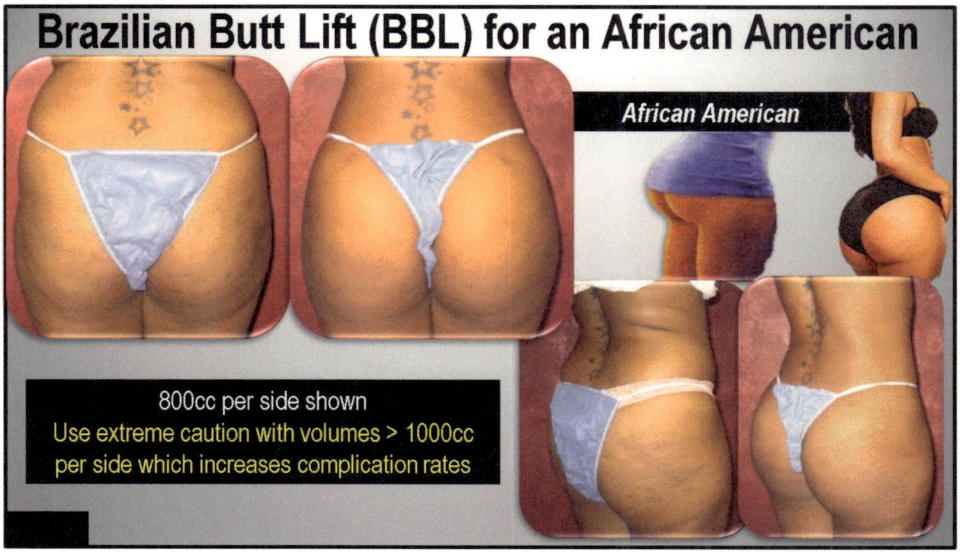

Figure 12.
BBLs for Latino / Hispanic women typically involves significant fat grafting to the mid and lower 1/3 of the buttock as well as major grafting in the lower lateral buttock. Even when a large implant is used, many Hispanic women will also want additional fill laterally with fat to accentuate the upside-down heart shape.

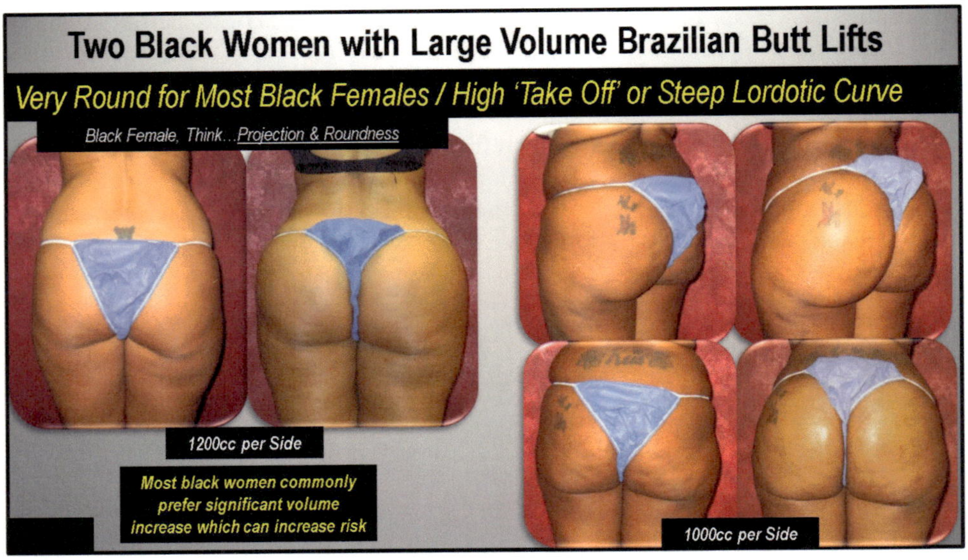

Figure 13.
Most Black females who desire BBLs have very consistent cultural request of a large, round buttocks that is almost "shelf-like" at the top. On average, women of this culture request a large, round buttocks with major fullness of the lateral buttocks and lateral thighs, as well as a substantial lordotic curve.

3. **Black female** patients have a very consistent cultural request of a very large and round buttocks (**Figure 12**). Another popular request in this ethnic group is a high "take-off" which is also known as a "shelf-like butt." In general, women of this culture request a very large, round buttocks with major fullness of the lateral buttocks and lateral thighs, and a major lordotic curve (**Figure 13**).

Of note, these ethnic variations are valid for most cases. However, interracial relationships may play a role in what patient's desire. Some Caucasian, Hispanic and Asian women may request the look of an African-American shape if they are in a significant relationship with an African-American male or if they socialize predominantly with that ethnic group. In a similar fashion, Black and Hispanic females in significant relationships with Caucasians may request reduction of the lateral thighs. Care must be taken to discuss details of what each individual patient hopes to achieve and what their specific preferences are regarding peri-gluteal shape and size.

4. Candidates for gluteal enhancements

As patients age, the buttock undergoes changing due to multiple factors including generics, gravity, weight gain and weight loss. The vast majority of patients experience fat hypertrophy in the peri-gluteal areas and a flattened buttock shape. One of the most important things for a surgeon is to categorize the patient based on their buttock shape. There are four major shapes identified. The "A" shape which the most desired shape as it typically follows the 0.7 waist-to-hip ratio. The "square" shape which is very common seen in those patients with excess waist circumference from increased adipose tissue around the waist and lower back region. The "O" shape is usually made up by a full and round buttock. Finally, the "V" shape buttock is often seen in the massive weight loss patient or in patients who have an atrophic buttock with excess fat adiposity in the "love handle" area (**Figure 4**). Another

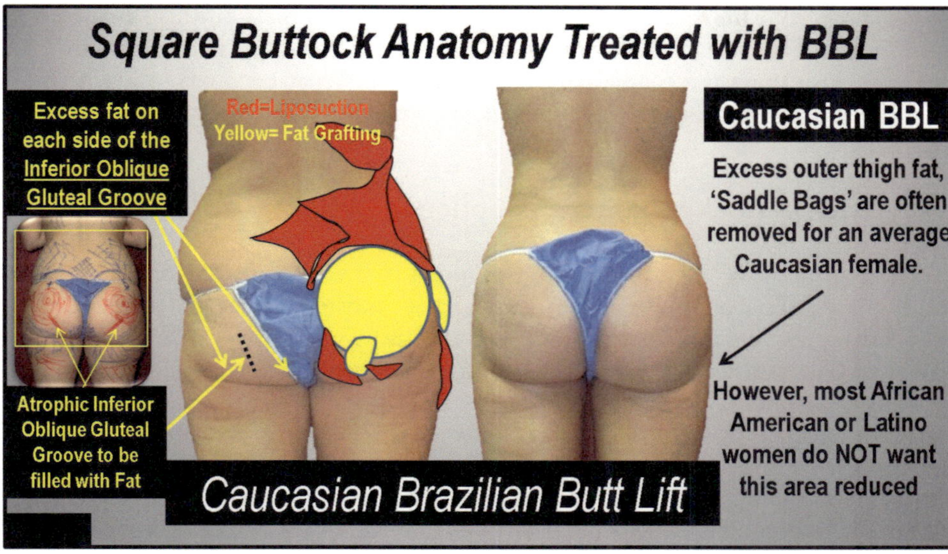

Figure 14.
A square buttock is very common and often is marked by a distinct inferior oblique groove that is observed in the lower pole and close to the medial third as shown There is usually excess fat on either side of the oblique groove. The square shape is mostly created from excess hip or flank fat.

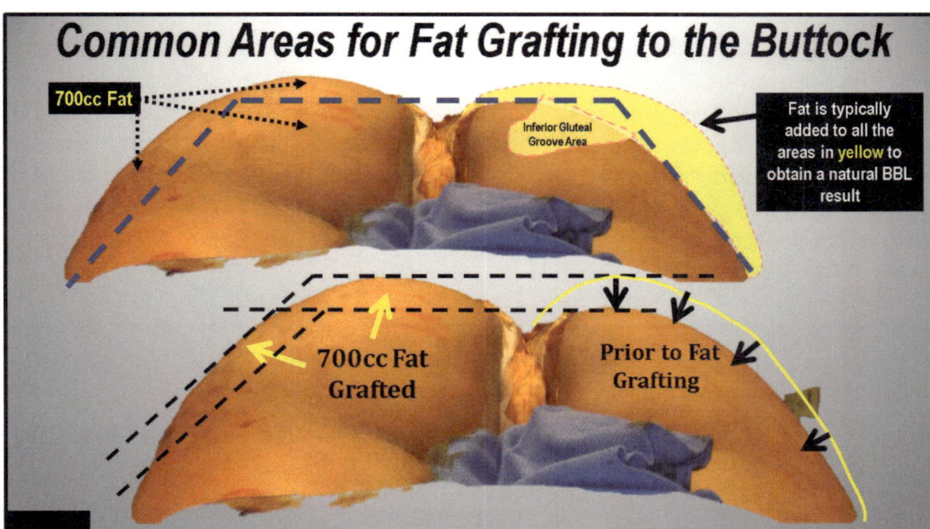

Figure 15.
Fat grafting should not be limited to the central buttock for best results. As shown, fat can be added to the oblique groove if present, posterior as well as lateral buttock and greater trochanter depression. Occasionally, fat may need to be blended even further down the patient's thigh.

remarkable finding is the inferior oblique gluteal crease that is most prominently seen in the "square" buttock (**Figure 14**). It is an oblique groove that is observed in the lower pole and close to the medial third. There is usually excess fat on either side of the oblique groove (**Figure 15**).

There are certain changes that take place in the gluteal and peri-gluteal region that take place over time which begin to change the buttock shape into a less ideal one. One of them is the loss of the inward curves at the level of the waist and also the inward sweep in the mid-line of the lower back (lumbosacral area). Another unaesthetic change of the aging buttock is the elongation of the infragluteal crease. One of the most aesthetic of a buttock is the "lifted" look which is why most buttocks that are considered attractive have their most prominent part in the upper to middle third. However, with aging and changes in weight, the buttock may become ptotic with most of its projection in the lower third and likely overhanging over the infragluteal crease.

5. Aesthetic buttock enhancement options

There are surgical and non-surgical therapies to correct deformities of the buttocks and to enhance its shape and size. The least invasive way to enhance gluteal deformities and irregularities is by injection of fillers such as poly-L-lactic acid (Sculptra by Galderma Laboratories, L.P.) which is a synthetic material that is naturally absorbed by the body over time. Sculptra® is indicated for healthy patients who are looking for correction of irregularities and small areas of atrophy. In the gluteal area is used off label since his FDA approval is for correction of facial wrinkles and deep nasolabial folds. The injection technique is considered subcutaneous to deep dermal in a cross-hatch pattern. It is recommended to ovoid overcorrection because the product is expected to gradually improve the contour deficiency after treatment of the area.

Surgical enhancement of the gluteal region depends largely on the amount of available fat to be harvested with liposuction and fat transfer. It also depends on the degree of skin laxity of the buttocks. Liposculpture (liposuction and fat transfer) is the preferred method of buttock augmentation on those female patients how have excess amounts of fat in the lower back, waist and/or abdominal area. This technique of liposculpture is popularly known and marketed as a "Brazilian butt lift" (BBL) procedure. The necessary amount of fat harvest needed varies on a case by case basis but on average 200–1000 cc of fat is micro-grafted into each side of the buttocks. In a recent reviewed survey of 100 board certified cosmetic surgeons who perform BBLs routinely, the average was 600 cc of fat inject per side. If the patient does not have enough excess fat available and is not willing to gain weight, then gluteal silicone implants are the treatment of choice (**Figure 16**).

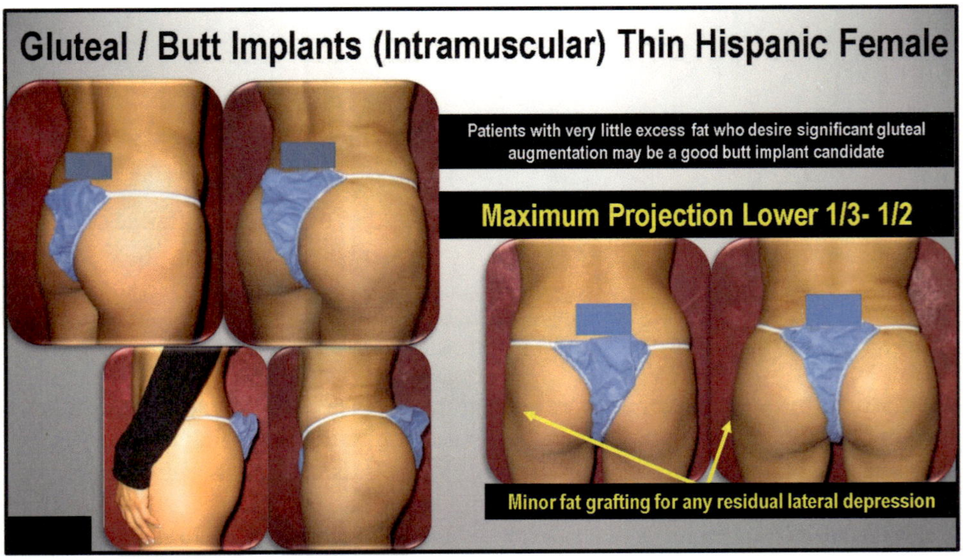

Figure 16.
Gluteal implants can be a great option for patients who desire significant gluteal enhancement but has very little excess fat. However, sometime even with implants, a Hispanic patient may want additional fullness laterally that can be performed simultaneously if at least some fat is available.

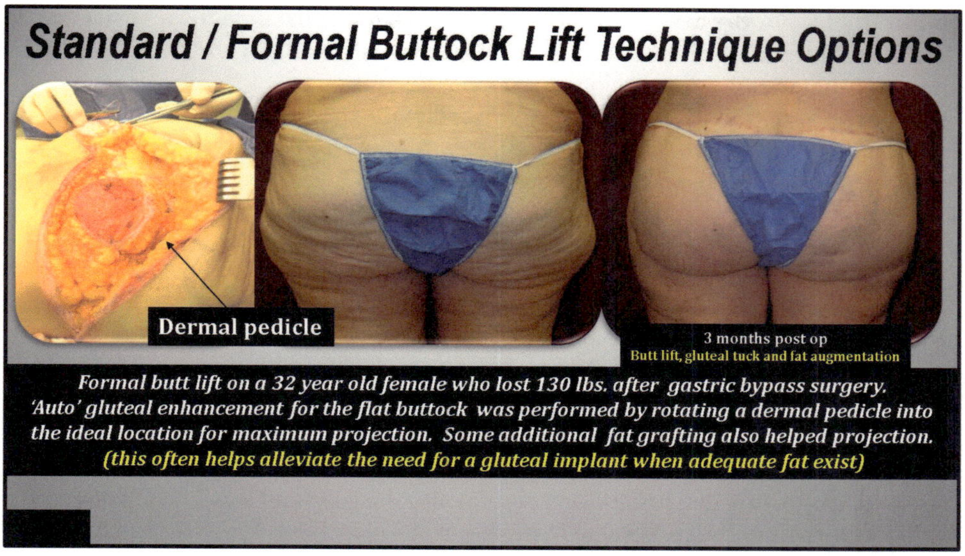

Figure 17.
In the massive weight loss patient with severe skin laxity, a traditional incisional butt lift is the treatment of choice. The enhancement in projection for those patients can be performed with auto-augmentation via use of a dermofatty pedicle as shown. Regrettably, it is limited to an isolated area and often additional fat injection laterally is required or implants if no extra fat source exist.

In the massive weight loss patient or patients with limiting amounts of fat and severe skin laxity, a traditional incisional butt lift is on treatment of choice. The enhancement in projection for those patients may be performed with micro-fat grafting and/or silicone gluteal implants (**Figure 17**). Auto-augmentation via use of a dermofatty pedicle during a formal butt lift adds bulk and projection, but unfortunately it is limited to an isolated area and often additional fat injection laterally is required or implants if no significant fat source exist.

The other type of patient that is often encountered is the patient that lacks projection in the gluteal region and desires an improved shape but are too thin for autogenous fat transfer. They usually have an athletic build and little to no gluteal ptosis. These patients have one option for aesthetic gluteal enhancement which is the surgical placement of a gluteal implant. Historically, one of the first ways surgeons started to augment the buttocks was with round silicone gel breast implants. However, surgeons quickly realized that breast implants were problematic in the buttock region [2]. Over the years, multiple techniques have been described for gluteal augmentation using prosthesis in three anatomical planes: submuscular, intramuscular and subfascial [3–5]. The submuscular placement is considered unfavorable because of the increased risk of injury to the sciatic nerve. This potential risk was minimized, but not eliminated, by placing the implant in an intramuscular plane. The subfascial technique virtually eliminates the morbidity of sciatic nerve injury but comes with other limitations such as a more visible and palpable implant.

6. Technical steps

6.1 Liposculpute technique (liposuction with autologous fat grafting, "Brazilian butt lift")

First, the fat donor sites are established. Common areas for fat harvest include, but are not limited to, the abdomen, chest, lateral thorax, waist, hips, back, arms, and/or thighs. For the best aesthetic outcomes, the lower back, sacrum, waist and hips are areas that are almost always treated with liposuction to narrow the waist and accentuate the curves and lower the hip/waist ratio.

Next, pre-surgical markings are preformed while the patient is in an upright position. Deep depressions or areas that need to be grafted are outlined in red and areas that need to be liposuction are marked in blue. Once the patient has been put under general anesthesia, foot pumps are applied for deep vein thrombosis prophylaxis and 2 g of cefazolin (Ancef) is given. If allergic to penicillin, clindamycin 600 mg IV is given as antibiotic prophylaxis.

Next, the skin is prepared in a sterile fashion with 4% chlorohexidine diluted with sterile 0.9% normal saline with sterile gauze to clean all areas that will be treated with liposuction or fat grafting. Then, a 20 gauge spinal needle connected to a Wells Johnson® infiltration pump is used to superficially inject the tumescent anesthesia solution. Next, a #11 blade is used to make punctures in all planned liposuction sites. Lastly, a blunt infiltration cannula attached to the infiltration pump is used to infiltrate with majority of the tumescent solution into the deep and superficial fat layers until the tissues have a tense feel to them due to the increase hydrostatic pressure. The tissues area left undisturbed for ~20 min to allow for vasoconstriction by the epinephrine within the tumescent anesthesia infiltrated. During this time, the patient is prepared and draped in a sterile fashion for a second time but this time using a ChloraPrep™ stick. In addition, a lap sponge soaked in betadine solution is placed and secured over the anus with one 3-0 prolene suture at the level of the sacrum and a 3 M ioband dressing to completely seal off the anus from potentially contaminating the sterile field (**Figure 18**). The maximum concentration of lidocaine used is 35 mg/kg and all cases are done under general endotracheal anesthesia.

Next, 3 or 4 mm liposuction cannulas are used to harvest the fat from all areas to be treated. The fat is collected sterile into a 3 L, glass, and reusable sterile canister. Excess fluid and blood settles on the bottom of the canister and fat micro-grafts float to the top of the canister via continuous vibration table. The excess fluid is decanted to isolate only the fat grafts. The fat is then treated with an antibiotic solution

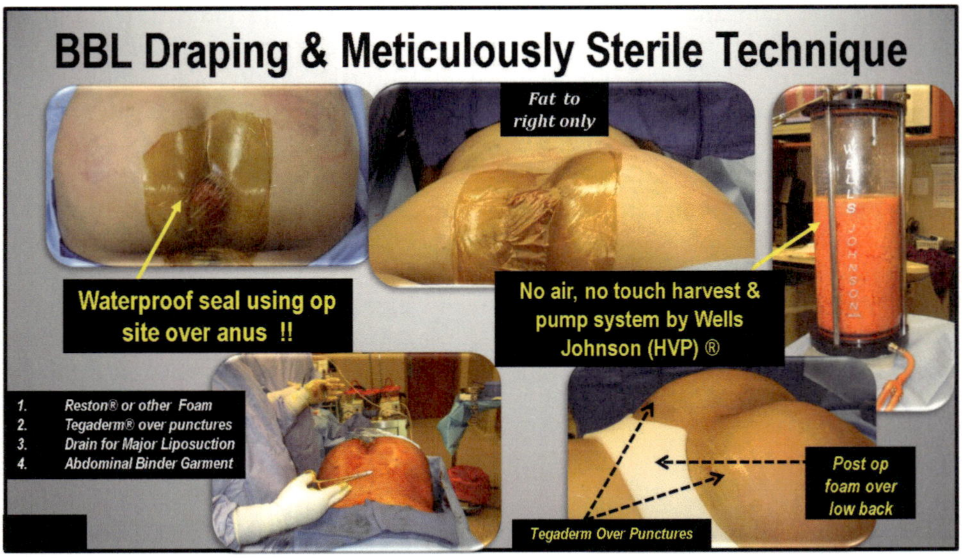

Figure 18.
A lap sponge soaked in betadine solution is placed and secured over the anus with one 3-0 Prolene suture at the level of the sacrum and covered with a 3M ioband dressing to completely seal off the anus from the sterile field. Drains are commonly used and punctures sealed sterilely in an effort to prevent post op infections.

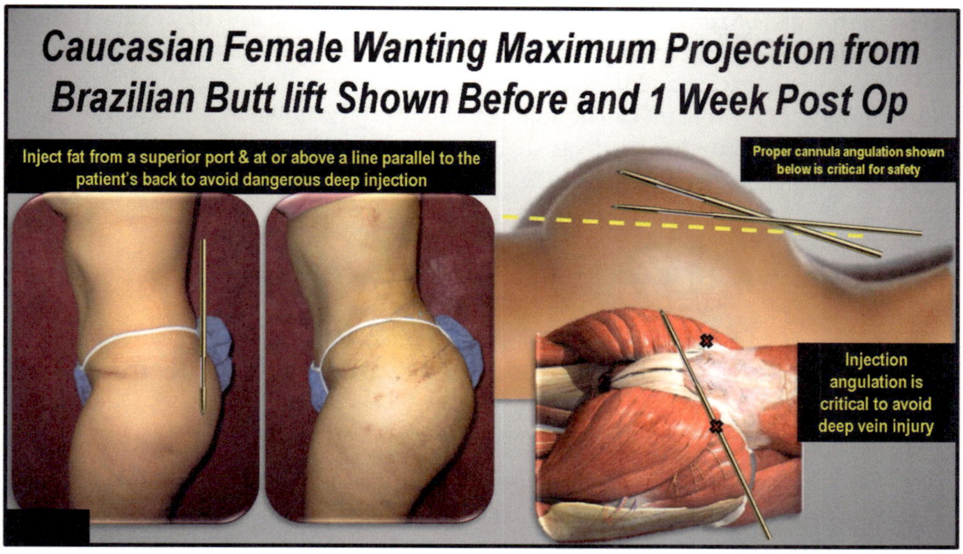

Figure 19.
The fat infiltration technique used by the authors is a superficial grafting technique above the muscle in a parallel plane to the back which keeps the cannula well above the superior and inferior gluteal veins. Injection should be keep out of the inner bowl of the pelvis and essentially stay above the boney crest.

containing 80 mg gentamicin and 600 mg of clindamycin mixed in a saline solution of 250 ml. Right before the fat is about to be injected back into the patient, 5–6 cc of platelet rich plasma (PRP) from the patient's own blood is mixed with the fat. A 4 mm infiltration cannula with a single hole is used to pump the fat back into the patient's buttocks. The fat infiltration technique most often used by the authors is a superficial grafting technique above the muscle in a parallel plane to the back and far from the superior and inferior gluteal veins to avoid injury which could lead to fat emboli (**Figure 19**). A pressure-controlled injection system by Wells Johnson is used which cuts off automatically if it senses pressures higher than central venous pressure. The preferred infiltration system is a closed loop injection system that includes a vibrating table to help with separation of the fat from the supernatant. The advantages of this system when compared to previous methods of fat grafting include efficiency, perfect micro-droplet size, more sterile or cleaner, and low pressure of injection.

6.2 Gluteal implants

First, the patient's upper and lower gluteal crease are marked. Then, the patient is asked to sit down to mark a horizontal line when the buttocks is touching the chair. The skin marking are made with a custom-designed template. The template fits perfectly into the gluteal area just above the horizontal line previously marked on the skin. Medial extend of the implant is ~2 cm lateral from the external rim of the sacral bone. Once the patient has been put under general anesthesia, foot pumps are applied for deep vein thrombosis prophylaxis and 2 g of cefazolin (Ancef) is given. If allergic to penicillin, clindamycin 600 mg IV is given as antibiotic prophylaxis.

Next, the skin is prepared in a normal sterile fashion and tumescent anesthesia is infiltrated into the sacral and gluteal areas. One single, vertically oriented, 6 cm incision is made in the midline of the sacral region in the intergluteal crease. The incision is made through skin, subcutaneous tissue and proceeds laterally until the lateral borders of the sacral bone and the medial border of the gluteal maximus is identified. A 4–6 cm incision is made intramuscularly blunt dissection is then performed intramuscularly laterally, caudally and in a cephalad direction to create the implant pocket.

This is performed bilaterally. The implants are then introduced into the pocket through the small incisions using a plastic funnel (**Figure 20**). The position of the implant is verified with palpation and the aesthetics of the augmentation is assessed from multiple angles. The implant can be adjusted slightly up or down to a limit. Often, a Latino female may want her implants slightly lower than what would be preferred by an African American female (**Figure 21**). Next, the implants are secure in place using a non-resorbable suture to the underlaying fascia. Layered closure is followed.

6.3 Formal incisional buttock lifting technique

As previously mentioned, this procedure is common in the massive weight loss patient. It is used to address the damage to collagen and elastic fibers which have been severely

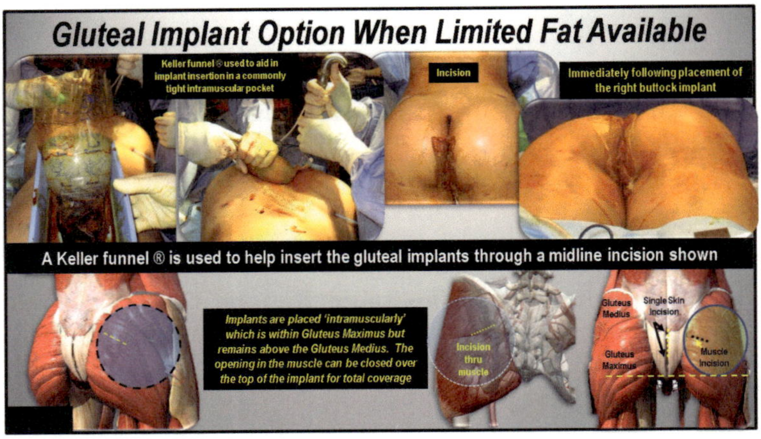

Figure 20.
A 5cm midline skin incision is used for placement of both butt implants followed by initial blunt dissection within the gluteus maximus muscle to create the implant pocket. After lighted retraction and hemostasis assured, implants are then introduced into the pocket through the small incisions using a Keller funnel®.

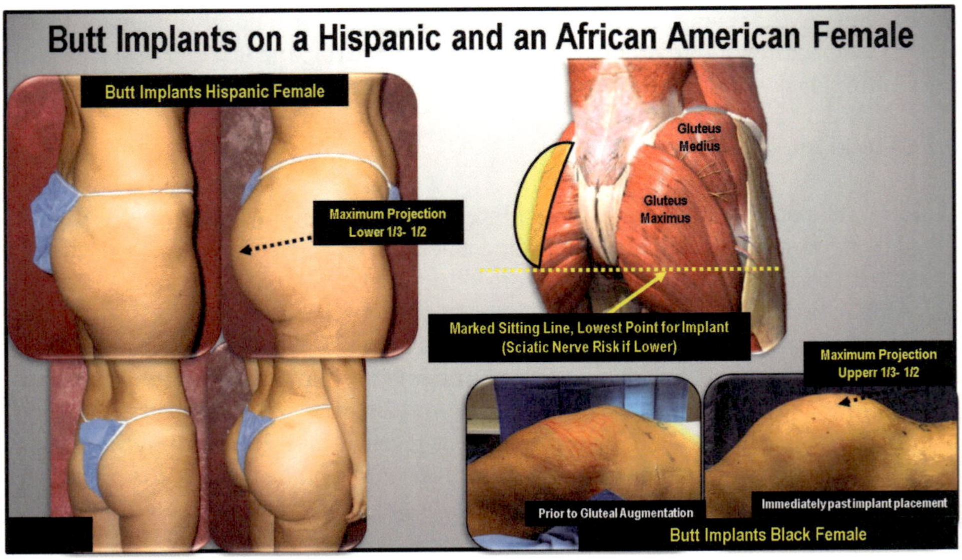

Figure 21.
The position of gluteal implants should be verified from multiple angles. After positioning, the muscle can be sutured primarily over the implant. Often, a Latino female may want her implants slightly lower than would be preferred by an African American female.

stretched. The typical "V" shape appearance of the massive weight loss patient is due to excess skin and lack of skin elasticity. The lack of projection is due to the loss of volume.

The incisional butt lift is a procedure that can be perfumed by itself to address the skin laxity and the ptosis of the skin. But it could also be combined with autogenous fat grafting and/or gluteal implants. The first step in this technique is to place the most superior incision along the iliac crest while the patient is standing in the upright position. This upper incision is marked from the mid-line and it ends laterally on the most lateral portion of the iliac crest. This creates a wide "M" shaped incision marking just above the underwear line. Then, a pinch test is performed in order to determine where the lower incision will be marked. The excess skin and fat excision is performed in a "Gull Wing" fashion (**Figure 22**). The patient is prepped and draped in a sterile fashion. Upper incision is made following the markings. No undermining above this incision is recommended. The only undermining of skin and subcutaneous

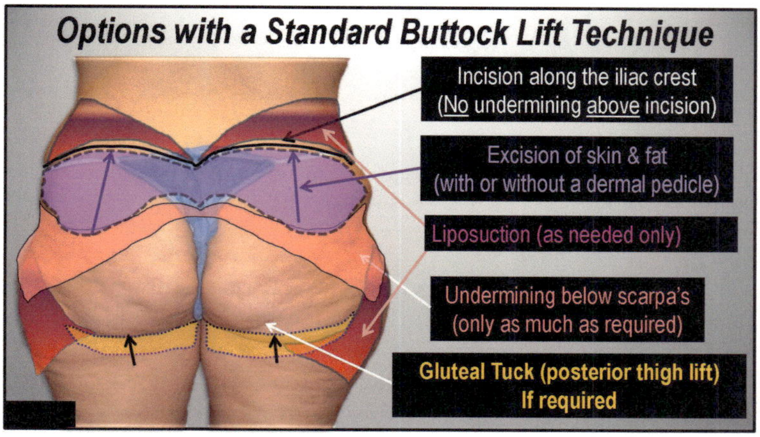

Figure 22.
The most superior incision for a formal butt lift is along the iliac crest while the patient is standing in the upright position. Then, a pinch test is performed in order to determine where the lower incision will be marked. The excess skin and fat excision is performed in a "Gull Wing" fashion. Minimal undermining is required and liposuction can be performed simultaneously along with occasional fat grafting or implants when indicated.

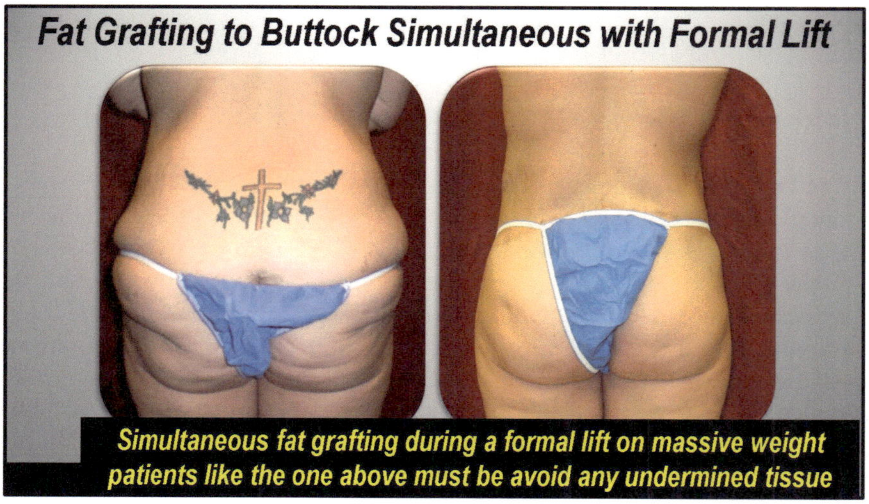

Figure 23.
The patient shown is before and after a standard skin excisional buttock lift with the addition of fat grafting to improve final shape and projection.

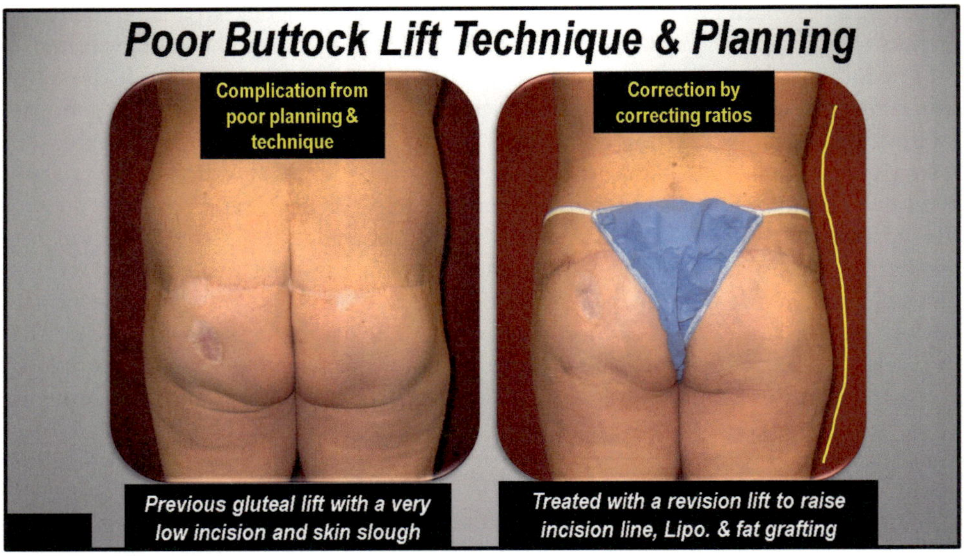

Figure 24.
The patient shown had complications from what appears to have been poor planning as well as technique. Correction focused on restoring a better hip to waist ratio by scar revision and fat grafting along with removal of fat at the true waist line.

fat is carried out in a caudal direction below Scarpa's fascia (**Figure 23**). Once the desired fat and skin has been excised, further undermining in a caudal direction takes place in order to be able to advance the lower skin and subcutaneous tissues up to the upper incision and close with the least tension as possible. Liposuction of the flanks and thighs is done only as needed. Another common procedural adjunct to an incisional but lift is a gluteal tuck which is also known as a posterior thigh lift.

In certain cases when fullness to the upper buttocks is desired, the surgeon should consider the rotation of a dermal pedicle inferiorly to give the upper buttocks more volume and projection. This could eliminate the need for a gluteal silicone implant. Planning is critical and one much keep correct proportions, maintain the superior incision at the iliac crest and avoid a thin flap to prevent unwanted complications (**Figure 24**).

7. Safety considerations

7.1 Infection prevention

Even though gluteal augmentation surgery has an incidence of infection of <1%, surgeons should avoid this serious complication at all cost. Patients should clean their entire body with an antiseptic skin cleanser the night before or the morning prior to surgery (i.e., Hibiclens® soap). All of our patient's get a double prep prior to surgery. One sterile prep takes place prior to tumescent or local anesthesia infiltration and the other prep takes places prior to incision time. Antibiotic prophylaxis with 2 g Ancef q4h, Unasyn 3 g q6h, and gentamicin 5 mg/kg/24 h [6]. In addition, the peri-anal area is also covered with a lap sponge soaked in betadine solution plus a seal over it using a 3 M™ Ioban™ adhesive intra-operatively, using a closed liposuction system for high volume fat harvesting and reinjection prevents the fat from ever being exposed to the open air in the operating room. Thus, reducing the risk for airborne pathogens. Prior to re-injection of fat, the harvested fat in the 3 L canister is treated with an antibiotic solution containing 250 cc of normal saline, 600 mg of clindamycin, and 80 mg of gentamicin. Lastly, all liposuction and injection punctures sites are sutured and sealed with sterile tegaderm dressings.

DOI: http://dx.doi.org/10.5772/intechopen.84660

7.2 Fat embolism prevention

Considered one of the rapidly evolving and one of the most popular cosmetic procedures of the last decades, the fat transferred procedure marketed as a "Brazilian butt lift" has been in the news in the past couple of years due to an increase in mortality rate associated to the potential risk for fat embolism and its fatal effect on the cardio-pulmonary system. In 2017, a report on mortality from gluteal fat grafting was published on the Plastics and Reconstructive Surgery Journal. The reports revealed that the mortality risk worldwide of 1:3000 for those patients undergoing gluteal fat grafting. Before that reports was published, the cosmetic surgery procedure associated with the highest mortality rate was attributed to abdominoplasty which is only 1:18,000. That makes the mortality risk for gluteal fat grafting six times higher when compared to abdominoplasty [7].

Fat embolism takes place when fat enters the venous system. Therefore, it is believed that fat is being grafted into the veins in the gluteal region and traveling up

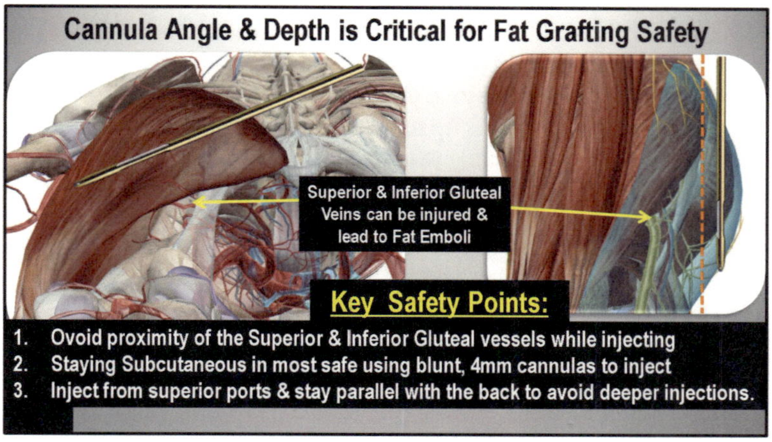

Figure 25.
Vascular injury and fat embolism into the superior and inferior gluteal vessels may be avoided by use of 4mm blunt cannulas and avoiding the use of smaller diameter cannulas that may more easily tear the vessels located deep to the gluteus maximus and medius.

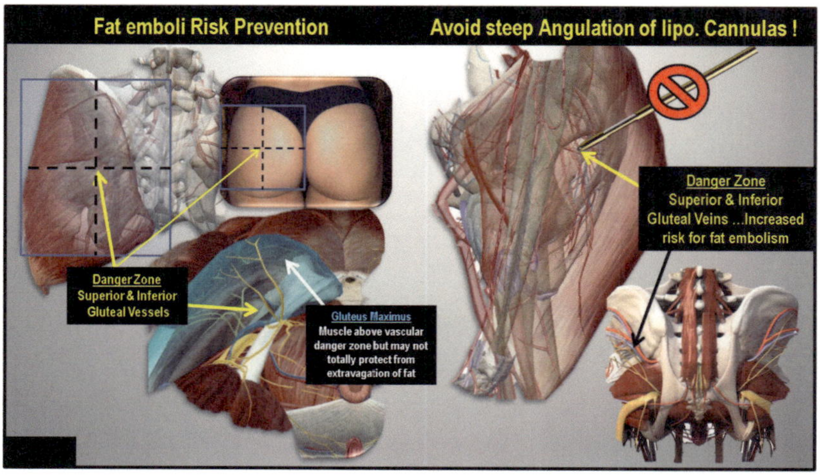

Figure 26.
The angulation of the infiltrating cannula is very important as shown. In order to avoid the "danger zone," it is suggested to keep the infiltration cannula as parallel as possible to the lower back and to resist angulating the cannula at a steep angle to avoid the deep gluteal veins.

into to cardio-pulmonary system. No one is aware of the exact mechanism but there are two theories. One is the "direct cannulation" theory, in which it is thought the cannula tip enters the vein and a bolus of fat is inserted into the vein. The fat bolus then can travel up to the pulmonary circulation and cause cardio-pulmonary instability. The second theory is the "laceration siphon" theory described by Del Vecchio and Wall [8]. In this theory, there is some iatrogenic damage to a large vein which is created under low pressure, which is then followed by fat introduction into the damaged vein under high pressure. It is thought that a pressure gradient in the area may transfer the fat slowly overtime into the damaged vein due to the difference in pressure. This theory has also been called the "Venous Traction" theory.

The evolution in technology used for large volume fat grafting are helping to make this procedure safer. The use of tommie-syringes for fat transferred is now considered outdated and somewhat high risk due to the variable and unpredictable amount of pressure needed to be applied to get the fat to come out. It is highly recommended to use a closed-circuit liposuction system in which the fat is kept sterile in a large cannister and then re-injected back into the patient without being exposed to air. The preferred system is the HVP™ system by Wells Johnson which allows you to precisely control pressure and flow rates. It allows you to manage and control both negative and positive pressures. The average positive pressure generated by a 60 ml Toomey syringe is 80″ Hg and a 1 ml syringe reaches up to 1425″ Hg. The standard infiltration pump that comes in the HVP™ system can create positive pressures up to 77″ Hg, and it allows you to set an upper limit so that the machine would automatically stop.

Another recommendation to ovoid vascular injury and fat embolism into the superior and inferior gluteal vessels is to use 4 mm blunt cannulas, avoiding the use of smaller diameter cannulas These vessels are located within the fascia or deep to the fascia of the gluteus maximus (**Figure 25**). Therefore, intramuscular injection of fat is not recommended and/or needed in order to achieve an aesthetic result. However, if the surgeon is going to inject fat into muscle, it is recommended to stay in the superficial portion of the muscle that is part of the convexity at or above the hip bone level, avoiding any deep muscle injection. It is also recommended to inject fat using a micro-droplet technique rather than large pooling boluses of fat.

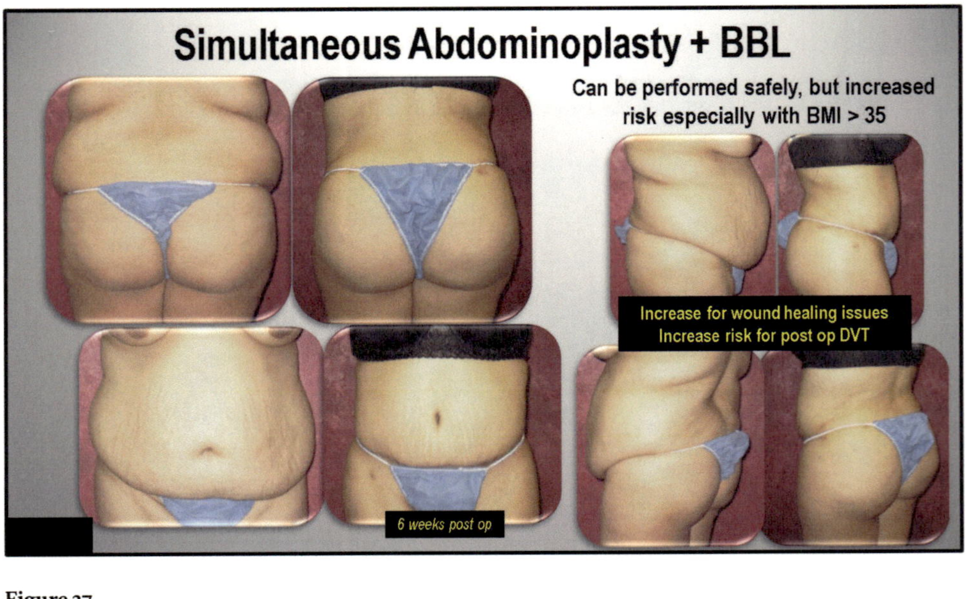

Figure 27.
A high risk obese patient is shown who underwent a simultaneous abdominoplasty plus liposuction and fat grafting BBL. A BMI >35 greatly increases her risk for many issues and especially wound problems.

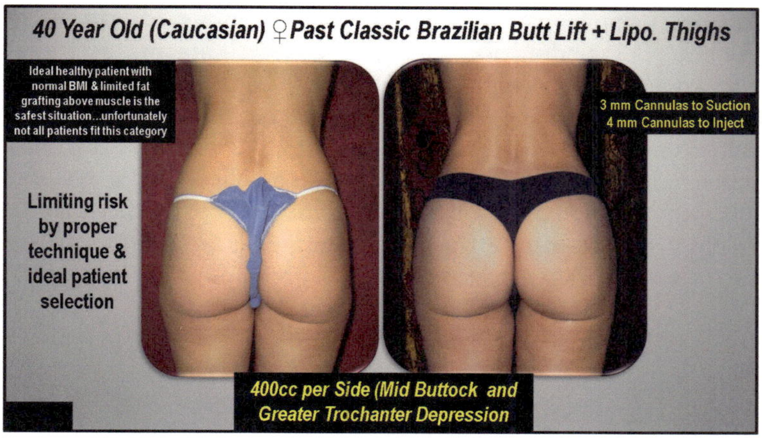

Figure 28.
Demonstration of the ideal patient for a BBL, healthy, normal BMI and limited fat volume injected above muscle to may a nice difference.

The angulation of the infiltrating cannula is also very important. In order to avoid the "danger zone," it is suggested to keep the infiltration cannula as parallel as possible to the lower back and to resist angulating the cannula in a steep angle (**Figure 26**). In addition, it is recommended to perform fat infiltration from the punctures made in the supra-gluteal crease which makes it less likely to inject fat intramuscularly than using the infra-gluteal crease.

7.3 Blood loss and DVT

Any of the main gluteoplasty procedures mentioned have the potential for heavy blood loss especially from aggressive liposuction. Patients with BMIs > 35 and those getting simultaneous abdominoplasty have increased risk of both anemia as well as deep venous thrombosis (DVT) (**Figure 27**).

We obtain pre and post-operative hemoglobin levels and hematocrit levels on all BBL patients as well as implant and formal butt lift patients. All patients have routine pneumatic foot pumps and other routine DVT prophylaxis. Lovenox, heparin or other anticoagulants are used on a case by case basis only since the risk for hematoma often outweighs the risk for DVT for many cosmetic surgery procedures, especially where major tissue undermining may be required (**Figure 28**).

8. Conclusions

Gluteal enhancement was a relatively infrequent procedure before the twenty-first century, but gluteal enhancement procedures have exploded in popularity after 2010 thanks mostly from social media and celebrities. Unfortunately, an unheralded increase in numbers of fat grafting procedures to the buttock throughout the world did not allow time for some complications to be realized in a timely manner. Many good surgeons around the world were caught off guard by this dangerous phenomenon. Fat embolism death has been associated with BBL procedures at an alarming frequency (mortality rate 1:3000). Fortunately, research and preventive measures are finally catching up and death rates from this procedure will expectantly fall precipitously in the next few years. This would be a welcome development to an otherwise excellent procedure. Many a patient have been thrilled with their ne shape and well-rounded curvy figure and small hip to waist ratio.

Beyond a BBL using fat, there are a multitude of options that can be used to improve the buttock including non-surgical injections, implants, excisional, liposuction and various energy devices. The surgeon must thoroughly understand the diagnosis to formulate the ideal plan and select the best technique for each patient. This chapter attempted to cover the top three surgical procedures (formal buttock lift, the Brazilian butt lift and gluteal implants) in enough detail to be very valuable for those performing these procedures. More than ever, the buttock plays a significant role in physical and sexual attraction and surgeons are ask routinely to obtain results that are beautiful as well as low risk.

Author details

Angelo Cuzalina[1*] and Armando Retana[2]

1 Tulsa Surgical Arts, Tulsa, Oklahoma, USA

2 American Board of Cosmetic Surgery, Chicago, Illinois, USA

*Address all correspondence to: angelo@tulsasurgicalarts.com

References

[1] Singh D. Adaptive significance of female physical attractiveness: Role of waist-to-hip ratio. Journal of Personality and Social Psychology. 1993;**65**:293-307

[2] Bartels RJ, Ó'Malley JE, Douglas WM, et al. An unusual use of the Cronin breast prosthesis. Case report. Plastic and Reconstructive Surgery. 1969;**44**:500

[3] Robles JM, Tagliapietra JC, Grandi MA. Gluteoplastia de augmento: Implante submuscular. Cirplast Ibero Latinoam. 1984;**10**:365-369

[4] Vergara R, Marcos M. Intramuscular gluteal implants. Aesthetic Plastic Surgery. 1996;**20**:259-262

[5] De la Pena JA. Subfascial technique for gluteal augmentation. Aesthetic Surgery Journal. 2004;**24**:265-273

[6] Roberts TL, Weinifeld AB, Bruner TW, Nguyen K. "Universal" and ethnic ideals of beautiful buttocks are best obtained by autologous micro fat grafting and liposuction. Clinics in Plastic Surgery. 2006;**33**(3):371-394

[7] Mofid MM, Teitelbaum S, Suissa D, et al. Report on mortality from gluteal fat grafting: Recommendations from the ASERF task force. Aesthetic Surgery Journal. 2017;**37**:796-806

[8] Del Vecchio D, Wall S. Expansion vibration lipofilling: A new technique in large-volume fat transplantation. Plastic and Reconstructive Surgery. 2018;**141**:639e-649e